Outsmarting Menopause

Outsmarting Menopause

Conversations about Metabolism, Muscles, Mood, and More

BROOKE BUSSARD, M.D.

Outsmarting Menopause:
Conversations about Metabolism, Muscles, Mood, and More

© 2025 Brooke Bussard

First Edition

Plants Over Animals, LLC

All rights reserved. No part of this book may be reproduced or transmitted in any form or by any electronic or mechanical means, including photocopy, recording, or any information storage and retrieval system, without prior written permission from the publisher, except by a reviewer, who may quote brief passages.

Content is not to be construed as medical advice. Consult your physician for matters regarding your personal health. The author is not liable for any damage allegedly arising from information in this book.

Editorial Services: Jetlaunch Publishing

Illustrations: Dorothy Windham

ISBN: 979-8-9877410-6-1 (hardcover)
ISBN: 979-8-9877410-4-7 (paperback)
ISBN: 979-8-9877410-5-4 (ebook)

This book is dedicated to all females.

Contents

Introduction | ix

1. HORMONES GO HAYWIRE Body Composition | 1
2. A THOUSAND SHEEP AND STILL COUNTING Sleep | 13
3. FASTING IS FOE FOR FEMALES Nutrition | 19
4. MUSCLES AFTER MENOPAUSE Strength Training | 31
5. HOLLOW BONES ARE FOR HUMMINGBIRDS Bone Health | 35
6. TO SIT OR NOT TO SIT Maximal Efforts | 49
7. FLEXIBLE FOR THE FUTURE Tendons and Ligaments | 59
8. SHOW ME THE SEROTONIN Mood | 65
9. THINK EXERCISE Brain Health | 73
10. HOT FLASHES AND HEART DISEASE Cardiovascular Health | 79
11. PINK FOR PREVENTION Breast Health | 87
12. ESTROGEN AFFECTS EVERYTHING Not So Obvious | 91

Bottom Line | 95

Frequently Asked Questions about Estrogen Supplementation | 97

Author's Note | 99

About the Author | 101

Contributors | 103

Introduction

Understanding and promoting health and wellness is a driving force in my life. I am passionate about helping people prevent, manage, and reverse disease. It's incredibly rewarding to see goals met and health measures improve.

However, there is a population where results are more challenging to obtain. Many women transitioning through menopause do not experience the results they deserve, despite their hard work and commitment. After much research, I realized that general health and fitness recommendations are missing crucial information for women in this specific stage of life.

When I entered the menopause transition, I suffered hot flashes and night sweats, along with episodes of fatigue. I discovered changes in my body composition (less muscle, more fat) despite my healthy diet and consistent exercise routine.

I refused to accept the changes were an inevitable result of aging and continued to look for more information. It turns out much of what women are told is based on research done with men—men whose bodies never experienced estrogen for several decades and then found themselves without it. However, I came upon new research looking specifically at menopausal women, and there are some critical differences between the sexes that influence the results.

Female hormones do more than help create life during reproductive years. Estrogen and progesterone regulate energy, mood, hunger, and so much more. And the effects of these hormones on the body are widespread—which is why women experience varied symptoms throughout each month for the decades we menstruate.

Females may feel energized at the beginning of a cycle when hormones are low, experience food cravings mid-cycle when progesterone surges, and suffer moodiness and bloating in the week before menstruation begins when hormones peak. All these symptoms are the result of hormonal shifts.

Once women reach perimenopause (the years leading up to menopause when the ovaries prepare for retirement), the hormones hop on a roller coaster and produce another round of symptoms. Overall, estrogen and progesterone levels fall, but they flail wildly like an inflatable air dancer outside a car dealership. The ratio of these two hormones fluctuates and causes internal stress and confusion. From the quintessential hot flash to the dysregulation of serotonin and everything in between, it takes a well-informed woman to make it through this stage of life feeling empowered.

Follow me on a journey to discover what happens as women transition through menopause. The stories in this book are based on real women and portray the struggles and the questions they have as they navigate this stage of womanhood. My goal is to shift the focus from dreading menopause symptoms to optimizing physical and mental health for the decades ahead.

Wishing you great health,

Brooke

1
HORMONES GO HAYWIRE

Body Composition

"What is going on with my midsection?" Shari shouts with annoyance. She's in her bedroom with two close friends, looking through her closet for an interview outfit.

Rachael chimes in, matching her friend's tone. "I'm having the same issue. My weight hasn't changed, but my pants are tighter around the waist, and it's very uncomfortable."

"My sister—who's a nurse—explained it to me," Ashley speaks up. "She says as we get older, we accumulate fat and lose muscle. Fat is less dense, so it takes up more space without moving the scale."

"Well, it's really irritating. How am I supposed to interview for a new job when none of my clothes fit?" Shari sits on the edge of the bed, her head in her hands. She is frustrated and on the verge of tears.

Ashley sits down and puts an arm around Shari's shoulders, "We'll figure it out. My sister says there's a lot of new information about menopause and how to manage it better."

"Could we treat her to lunch tomorrow and get her insights?"

"I'll text her." Rachael starts typing. "Yup, she's available. Noon at The Bistro."

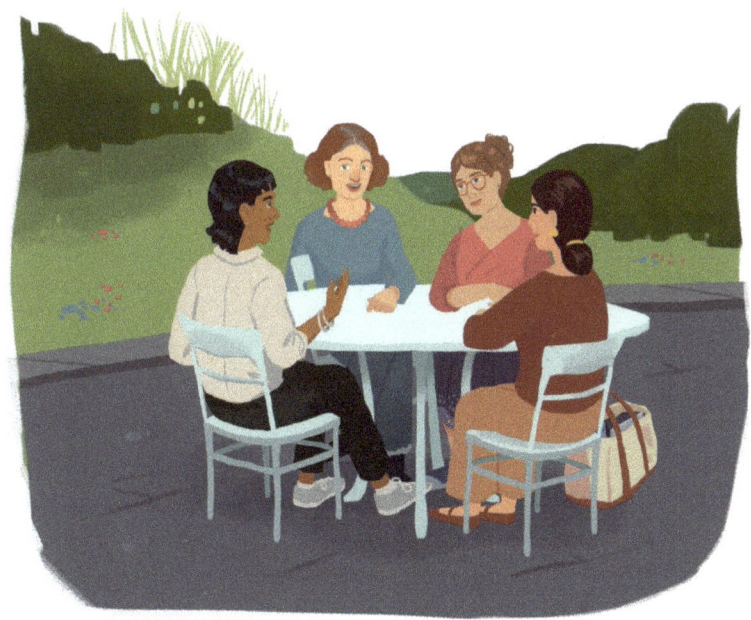

Ashley and her sister April join Rachael and Shari at an outdoor table overlooking the park. After a few family updates, April jumps right in, knowing an hour is never enough time to talk about menopause.

"I bet all three of you are in perimenopause," she says to Ashley and her friends. "Women in their forties are at the mercy of fluctuating hormone levels as the body gets closer and closer to menopause. And the symptoms can vary a lot—headaches, joint pain, anxiety, forgetfulness, not to mention the typical hot flashes and night sweats."

Rachael interrupts, "What's the difference between menopause and perimenopause?"

"Menopause marks one day in time. It's the day one year from your last period.

"Perimenopause includes the years leading up to menopause when the ovaries start to shut down. The span of time varies for each woman, but the average is around four years. For some, it's much shorter, and for others, it can last a decade," April explains.

What is menopause?

Technically, it's the day when a woman has not had a period for a year. The menstruation is officially paused. (Actually, it ended, but we don't call it "menoend".)

The average age for natural menopause is 51, with the normal range being 45 to 55. Perimenopause can begin a decade before the last menstrual cycle, and hormones—estrogen and progesterone—fluctuate erratically throughout those years. Those fluctuations create the many symptoms we associate with menopause.

Some women go through menopause earlier, particularly if they smoke, live at high altitudes, or have certain medical conditions. Cancer treatments, surgery, and other medical therapies are common causes of early menopause. Later menopause happens for some women who have more children, use oral contraceptives, or have a higher body mass index.

Regardless of the reason or timeframe, menopause is the start of life in an altered hormonal environment. Learning how to flourish under the new conditions is paramount to thriving in the postmenopausal years.

"During our reproductive years—from the time we get our first period until we start perimenopause in our thirties or forties—our hormones work in harmony like a great a cappella group."

A Closer Look at Hormones during the Reproductive Years

Let's review the hormonal cycle of the reproductive years.

After the female body goes through the turbulence of puberty, it settles into an undulating and fairly predictable cycle of estrogen and progesterone for several decades.

The normal menstrual cycle happens roughly every 28 days but can be shorter or longer for various reasons. The "spectrum of normal" is 21 to 40 days.

The cycle involves signals sent from the brain to the ovaries to release hormones that encourage reproduction through the following events:

1. Estrogen levels rise for about two weeks, causing the release of an egg.
2. The egg travels down the fallopian tube to the uterus.
3. Progesterone rises, causing the uterine lining to thicken and become a cozy place for a fetus to grow.
4. If the egg is not fertilized, both estrogen and progesterone levels drop, and the uterine lining is shed as a period.

Cycles vary the most in the first five to seven years after periods start and during the last ten years before the periods end.

April continues, "During perimenopause, estrogen and progesterone levels decline but not in a linear fashion. They fluctuate up and down. Also, the ratio of the two hormones changes. Sometimes there is an overload of estrogen compared to progesterone, and at other times, the level of estrogen is relatively low in relation to progesterone. These two factors, the change in the levels plus the change in the ratio, create stress in the body."

"And stress causes us to gain weight?" Shari asks as she points to her midsection.

"Yes. Stress from internal sources—like fluctuating hormones—or external sources—like a big project at work—generates the release of cortisol. And cortisol causes the body to store fat."

"Why would it do that?" Rachael wonders.

April explains, "Cortisol not only helps with an immediate stress response, it also prepares for future stress. It promotes fat storage to ensure energy needs can be met."

"So, the hormonal changes cause stress inside the body, resulting in the release of cortisol. Cortisol makes us store fat. Stored fat is causing me stress. Sounds like a vicious cycle," Shari adds, her voice tinged with worry.

April replies, "It can be. During the decades when our hormones cycled in a predictable way, the body knew what to expect. But with changing levels of hormones during the menopause transition, we need to find other ways to restore equilibrium between the two sides of our nervous system, the 'fight or flight' and the 'rest and digest.'" She moves her left palm up and lowers her right one to demonstrate finding balance between the sympathetic and parasympathetic nervous system.

The Role of Cortisol

Cortisol is a hormone critical for survival. Typically, the adrenal glands that sit on top of each kidney release a pulse of cortisol in the morning to help regulate blood sugar, blood pressure, and metabolism. Cortisol levels fluctuate throughout the day in response to activity, but generally, the level is highest in the morning and lowest at night before bedtime.

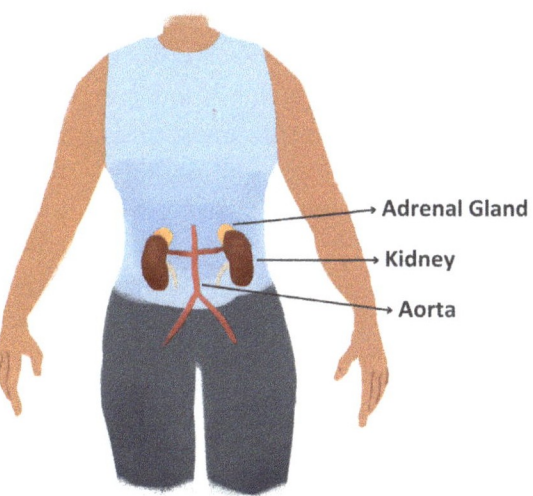

Think of cortisol as the maestro of metabolism. Cortisol mobilizes resources in response to stress, telling the body to increase heart rate and deliver more oxygen and glucose to cells.

Because almost all tissues in the body have receptors for cortisol, it affects everything, including the immune system, the cardiovascular system, and the musculoskeletal system.

Consistently high levels of cortisol can have negative effects on your health, but levels that are too low can be detrimental as well.

Rachael thinks about a recent conversation with another friend, "Can't we just take HRT?"

"HRT, hormone replacement therapy, or MHT, menopause hormone therapy, involves adding estrogen back into the system. This can help dampen some of the symptoms like hot flashes, but it can't turn back the clock and recreate the environment your body was used to. For one thing, there are fewer receptors for estrogen to bind to as we get older. We need to adjust our lifestyle to help us maintain a healthy weight and avoid the extra pounds from sneaking up on us."

The waiter stops at their table and asks if they'd like anything else. They decline as Rachael reaches for a fry on April's plate.

"Does cortisol make you eat more? I feel like I am always hungry—like when I used to take a Medrol dose pack when my asthma flared up," Rachael asks.

"Definitely. Cortisol and Medrol are both steroids that increase your appetite and cravings, especially for sugar and fat. Steroids also break down muscle tissue and lower metabolism to save energy. It's part of the body's survival mechanism."

"Did you say cortisol *lowers* metabolism?" Rachael is incredulous.

"It does, but indirectly. When cortisol is elevated for longer periods of time, it breaks down muscle tissue. Because muscle uses a lot of energy, our metabolism is lower when we have less of it."

"And, when cortisol levels stay elevated, your cells don't respond well to insulin. Without insulin, glucose can't get into cells to be used for fuel, so the body stores the sugar as fat, especially around the midsection."

"Go figure," Shari mumbles.

"Here's where it gets a little more complicated," April continues. "Belly fat comes in two varieties. Subcutaneous fat is found just under the skin. It's the fat we grab when we 'pinch an inch.'

"Visceral fat is found further inside the body around organs and accumulates when cortisol and insulin levels go awry. This type of fat causes inflammation and is linked to chronic diseases like obesity, heart disease, diabetes, and cancer."

"How do we know which kind of fat we have?" Shari asks.

"Measure your waist-to-hip ratio. Find the narrowest part of your waist and divide it by the widest part of your hips, where your butt is the biggest; if the number is over 0.85, you probably have too much visceral fat."

"How do we get rid of it?" Shari sits up straight, putting her hands on the sides of her waist.

"The body will store less fat if we can reduce the chronically elevated cortisol level. That's where exercise and sleep can be helpful. And, of course, nutrition. Foods that fight inflammation are especially helpful."

Shari leans in. "Which foods are those?"

"Unprocessed whole plant foods, including fruits, veggies, beans, and whole grains, contain nutrients that can stop inflammation. Think of these foods as a medicine you can take several times a day. If they had a flashy label and a snazzy description of their benefits, people would definitely buy them!"

Shari takes a minute to process all this new information. "Will these foods help me get rid of this fat?"

"Yes, but remember, some amount of body fat is normal and necessary. It's the *excess* body fat that leads to chronic diseases."

"What's a normal percentage of body fat?" Rachael asks.

"It depends on a number of factors including body type, age, and ethnicity, but mid to upper twenties is generally considered healthy during perimenopause and postmenopause."

"Oh, that's higher than I would have guessed," Ashley interjects.

"Yeah, but the average woman is actually around 34 percent."

April elaborates, "Many women calculate their BMI—body mass index—and if it's in the normal range, they assume they're healthy. But they could still be obese based on body fat percentage."

"Is that what 'skinny fat' means?" Rachael wonders aloud.

"Sure. That's another way to say 'normal weight obesity'. A woman may weigh the same amount her whole life, but as she ages and loses bone and muscle mass, the amount of fat in her body increases. The average woman loses thirteen pounds of lean mass—bone and muscle—between the ages of twenty-five and sixty-five.

"If you swap those thirteen pounds of muscle and bone for fat, it can dramatically change your body composition," Ashley says emphatically.

BMI: A Useful Tool, But Not the Whole Story

Body mass index (BMI) looks at the ratio of height to weight to estimate body fat. It's a quick and inexpensive way to categorize a body as underweight, normal, overweight, or obese.

BMI is a useful tool for identifying weight categories that may be associated with health problems, but it's not necessarily an accurate representation of someone's true health status.

For example, athletes with high lean muscle mass can be categorized as overweight or obese according to their BMI. But in fact, their body fat percentage is low.

In the case of postmenopausal women, they can carry too much fat even when their weight is in a normal range for their height, making their BMI deceivingly low.

"How can we figure out our body fat percentage?" Ashley says as she starts to search on her phone.

"DEXA scans are a great way, and you can get it done at the same time as your bone density test. But there are other devices in doctors' offices and fitness centers to measure body fat."

"Are you talking about the InBody scans?" Shari asks.

"Yeah, they use a method called bioelectrical impedance analysis, or BIA. An electrical current goes through the body. You don't feel it at all," April explains as Shari's face scrunches. "The currents move at different rates through water, fat, muscle, and other tissue to determine body composition."

April's phone rings just as the waiter brings the check. Ashley signals to April that she can take off because the ladies are paying for her lunch. April nods to everyone as she leaves the table.

The ladies say their goodbyes and head back to their cars.

As Shari and Rachael walk together, Shari shakes her head. "I knew it was more complicated than just 'calories in, calories out.' I've tried eating 900 calories a day—or less—and still don't lose weight." She furrows her brow, thinking about high cortisol, slow metabolism, and inflammation.

As they hop into the car, Rachael glances at Shari. "So… does that mean skipping meals to lose weight is a bad idea?"

"I think so. It sounds like starving yourself just leads to muscle loss, weaker bones, and, honestly, feeling miserable. The real focus should be lowering cortisol."

"Got it. Fix the root cause. I just read an article this morning that said sleep can help lower cortisol."

GLOW BOWL FROM THE BISTRO

SERVES: 4   PREP TIME: 35 MINUTES

INGREDIENTS:

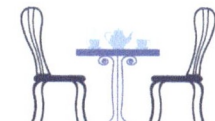

1 cup cooked green lentils
1 cups cooked quinoa
2 cups sweet potatoes, cubed
2 cups broccoli, chopped
A handful of baby spinach or arugula
1 avocado, sliced
Pickled red onions (optional garnish)
Toasted pumpkin seeds or almonds for crunch

Lemon-Tahini Drizzle
1/2 cup tahini
2–3 tbsp lemon juice
1 garlic clove, minced
1–2 tbsp warm water (to thin)
Salt and pepper to taste
Optional: a touch of maple syrup or Dijon mustard

DIRECTIONS:

Preheat oven to 400 F. Spread sweet potatoes on baking tray lined with parchment paper. Roast for 15 minutes, then flip potatoes, add broccoli to the tray and roast for another 15 minutes.

Assemble bowls: Start with a base of quinoa and greens. Arrange 1/2 cup of lentils, 1/4 of the roasted veggies, and 1/4 of the avocado around each bowl. Drizzle generously with lemon-tahini sauce. Top with pickled onions and toasted seeds for crunch.

2
A THOUSAND SHEEP AND STILL COUNTING

Sleep

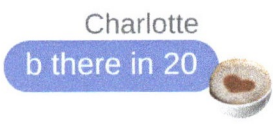

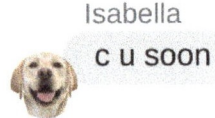

Charlotte rushes into the meeting room where other volunteers are preparing items for the school auction. "Sorry I'm late. I finally fell asleep around three and didn't hear my alarm."

Isabella commiserates, "I hear you. I can't remember the last time I got a good night's sleep."

Jill rolls her chair over from the neighboring table. "Just another great gift from Mother Menopause. Well, maybe not for you, Hazel." She waves off the younger mom.

"Why does menopause make it hard to sleep?" Charlotte bemoans.

Hazel speaks up. "I'm a physician's assistant for a gynecologist, and we see patients with sleep issues every day, *especially* as they approach menopause. The decline in estrogen and progesterone levels can make a mess of things."

Jill is surprised. "Tell us more!"

"Estrogen plays a role in sleep," Hazel explains. "It helps you fall asleep quickly, decreases the number of times you wake up, and increases total sleep time and quality. And progesterone helps to relax the body."

"What are we supposed to do when we don't make those hormones anymore?" Isabella asks.

"You need a sleep routine," Hazel replies.

"What do you mean?" Jill asks.

"Basically, go to bed and wake up at the same time every day. And you might need a plan to wind down before bed, like reading or listening to music." Hazel starts sorting through a bag of small donations.

"How much sleep should I get?" Isabella inquires.

"We tell our patients to sleep from ten at night to six in the morning." Hazel tosses a pack of fluffy socks to Isabella to add to one of the baskets. "It will help you sync up with your natural circadian rhythm," Hazel offers.

"I always enjoy the quiet hours in the house when everyone's asleep. That's going to be hard for me," Charlotte announces with slight disgust.

"Then try to go to bed thirty minutes earlier each week until you can get your bedtime between ten or eleven."

"Anything else we can do?" Isabella chuckles as she tosses a bright floral bathrobe to Jill. It looks expensive but is clearly not her taste.

Hazel replies, "Ditch the screens before bed, including your phone. The blue light stimulates the brain and suppresses melatonin production making it harder to wind down."

"I love scrolling Insta before bed. Can I take a melatonin supplement instead?" Isabella asks.

"You can, but it's always better if the body provides hormones naturally."

"What about dinner? I've heard eating close to bedtime can interfere with sleep, but I eat late because the kids have band and soccer practice after school." Jill lets out a sigh.

"Ideally, you should eat dinner a few hours before you go to bed so your body can rest and recover during sleep. If the body is still digesting food, it's harder to reach the deeper stages of sleep."

"Sometimes I wake up hungry, though," Charlotte says.

"Hmm, you may be under-fueled. Being in a calorie deficit can also affect sleep. Look at your total calories and the quality of your calories." Hazel holds up a very trendy necklace. "I'm bidding on this!"

"When I have a rough night, I'm so hungry the next day," Isabella adds.

"When we're sleep-deprived, the hormones that regulate appetite—ghrelin and leptin—become unbalanced. This makes it harder to feel full and to control food intake. So a poor night's sleep can lead to overeating the next day." Hazel puts a bow on a finished basket as she talks.

Hunger & Fullness: How Hormones Control Appetite

Ghrelin and leptin are hormones that work in opposition to each other to regulate hunger and energy storage.

Ghrelin, known as the Hunger Hormone or growlin' ghrelin, stimulates appetite and makes you hungry.

Leptin, known as the Satiety Hormone, taps the brakes on appetite and makes you feel full.

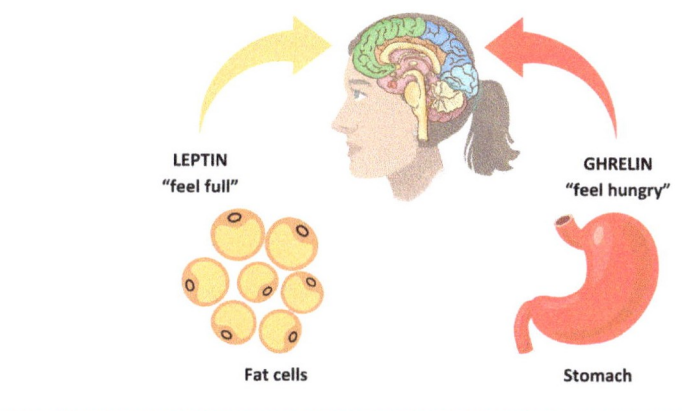

Jill chimes in, "My big complaint is the lack of energy from sleepless nights. I don't feel like exercising, and even if I drag myself to the gym, I feel sluggish and wonder if I'm wasting my time."

"It's not easy to sync all the pieces—exercise, sleep, and nutrition—because they all impact each other. Try setting smaller manageable goals each day to slowly make progress in each area.

"Start with an extra fifteen minutes of sleep and a small amount of exercise. In time, you'll reach your goal without feeling overwhelmed." Hazel's tone is upbeat and encouraging.

She adds, "And if you are lying in bed not sleeping, stay there. Don't get anxious about falling asleep. Even when you are resting your body, there's a benefit.

"It may take weeks to months for the sleep efforts to start showing results. So be patient; it will be worth it. While you sleep, the body produces growth hormone, which is important for building muscle, burning fat, and recovering from workouts. And growth hormone helps lower cortisol, the stress hormone." Hazel adds another scented candle to the growing collection.

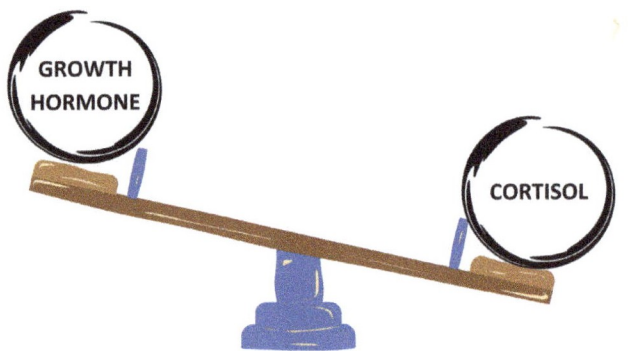

Growth Hormone Up, Cortisol Down

"So, if I get more sleep, I'll have a better recovery from my workouts?" Jill starts assembling a basket with a goodnight theme—lavender-scented bath salts, a sleep mask, and a white noise machine.

"Absolutely, and even more so if you can get to bed earlier. Growth hormone secretion is tied to our circadian rhythm and peaks during the early stages of deep sleep. If you're asleep by ten, this occurs around midnight. Add a cute pen and notepad set to the goodnight basket." Hazel reaches across the table and hands them to Jill.

"Why are you adding those?" Charlotte wonders aloud.

"For the busy brains at bedtime. You know, when thoughts race around in your head when you're trying to sleep. If you write them down, the brain can relax and allow you to drift off."

Hazel glances at her watch. "I've got to head to work, but I'll text you some other suggestions."

Hazel

Sleep tips! And if hot flashes wake you up, read through that section too.

HEALTHY SLEEP HABITS
- **Consistent Bedtime and Wake time**
- **Screens Off**
- **Pen & Paper on bedside table**
- **No food for 2 hours before bed**
- **No alcohol for 1 hour before bed**
- **Be mindful of caffeine**
- **Block out light and noise**
- **Stay cool**

HOT FLASH RELIEF
- **Breathable, moisture-wicking sheets like cotton or bamboo**
- **Gel pillows, cooling mattress pad, or cold pack near your neck or wrists**

3
FASTING IS FOE FOR FEMALES

Nutrition

Caroline and Claire navigate life together. Since the day they were born, their mother has been in awe of the twins' unwavering bond. At 46, the siblings still hold hands when walking down a sidewalk.

They eat healthy foods and include a variety of fruits and vegetables in their meals. They watch their portion sizes, but both of them have recently gained weight and can't figure out why.

"What is going on?" Caroline says under her breath as she tries on a few hand-me-downs from Claire, who is constantly revamping her wardrobe.

"Well, I'm glad it's not just me. I couldn't button those either." Claire would never give Caroline those jeans if they still fit. They were her favorite pair and a huge splurge that had paid for themselves in years of frequent wear and boosted confidence.

"I heard Jada talking about intermittent fasting. Maybe we should ask her about it. If it's working, we could try it to lose a few pounds." Caroline picks up her phone and starts texting.

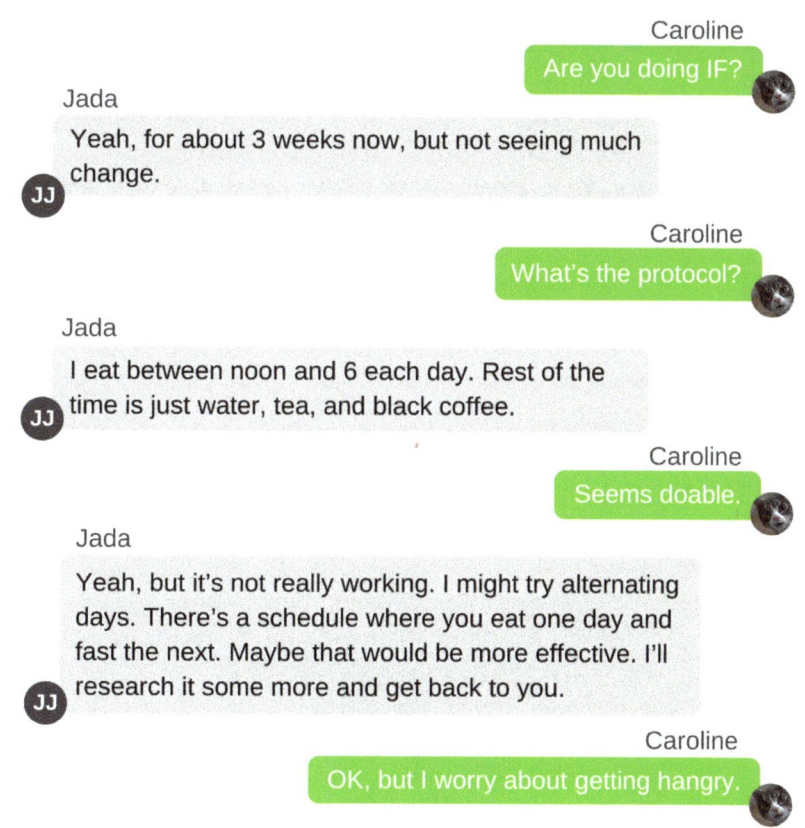

Later that day, Jada shows up at Caroline's townhouse. Claire is doing laundry since her new washer won't be delivered for a few days.

"Well, it's a good thing I did more research," Jada exclaims. "It turns out women shouldn't fast! That's the last time I blindly follow Jim's routine."

Claire is confused. "Aren't fewer calories always helpful to lose weight?"

"Sure, but fewer is relative," Jada explains. "You lose weight if calories-in are less than calories-out. But it's not simple or straight-forward. For example, two people can eat the same number of calories, but one person might absorb fewer calories than the other person."

Claire asks, "Why?"

"If they have inflammation in their digestive tract, like with IBS—irritable bowel syndrome—or Crohn's disease, less of the food gets digested. That's one of many possible reasons."

Caroline adds, "Doesn't the microbiome also affect absorption?"

"It does," Jada replies. "The types and amounts of bacteria in your gut affect how food is broken down and absorbed."

"And what about the calories-out piece of the puzzle?" Claire answers her own question. "I guess that changes based on body size. I know I burn fewer calories than Curt when we hike the same distance and time."

"Yeah, and there are other factors that influence our metabolism," Jada says. "The bottom line is that it's complex.

"And it's even more complicated for women. When the female brain senses a calorie deficit—particularly when it expects fuel—it treats it as stress. This triggers cortisol release, decreases the production of thyroid hormones, and slows metabolism."

"Making the calories-out part of the equation smaller," Caroline follows along.

"Right, and the body adapts to having less food," Jada adds.

"Okay, so what's the answer? What should we do?" Caroline says with both palms in the air.

Jada replies, "First, make sure your brain knows there is enough energy for normal metabolism. We don't want the body to slow down because it thinks there is famine in the forecast."

"How?" Claire asks.

"Focus on timing. Let your body know it has fuel when it needs it, especially first thing in the morning."

"Can I drink my dark roast in the morning and split my calories between lunch and dinner?" Caroline loves her coffee and refills three or four times before noon.

"No!" Jada says emphatically. "When you wake up, let the body know fuel is on the way. Cortisol levels spike within a half hour of waking. Providing the body food prevents the cortisol levels from staying elevated, and it sends a note to the brain saying, 'Don't worry about searching for food today.'"

She adds, "If you don't love breakfast, keep it light but give your body something to lower the cortisol level."

The women discuss breakfast options.

"I'm good with peanut butter on toast or overnight oats with apples and cinnamon—those Cosmic Crisp apples are *so* good right now!"

"I always love a smoothie."

"You should try the breakfast cookies Jim's sister makes. They're *amazing*! I'll send you the recipe."

"But how many calories should we eat?" Claire asks.

"It depends on age, activity level, and a lot of other factors. It's important to get enough fuel to keep the body running, like keeping your heart beating, your digestive system moving, and all the other stuff going on in the body, plus provide fuel for the activities of the day," Jada explains.

"The average woman probably uses about 1,400 calories per day before counting exercise. But remember, everyone is different, and you need to make adjustments to figure out what works for you."

"Wow, that's way more than I thought. What should we do if we want to lose a few pounds without our cortisol going up?" Caroline turns back to Jada to figure out how to solve this puzzle.

"Reduce calories at the end of the day. Stop eating two or three hours before bed to cut out a few hundred calories."

"I already don't eat after dinner," Claire responds with concern.

"Try decreasing the portion size of your dinner or swap some foods so the caloric density is lower. Eat foods with lots of fiber and water, like steamed vegetables; those foods have fewer calories per pound, and you should still feel full."

Claire gives Jada a look that says, 'Tell me more.'

"It's all about calorie density. For example, compare an apple and a block of cheese. The apple has 237 calories per pound because it is filled with water and fiber. Cheese, on the other hand, is calorically dense with 1,871 calories per pound. I'll text you a calorie density chart."

"Thanks!"

Jada
Here you go! JJ

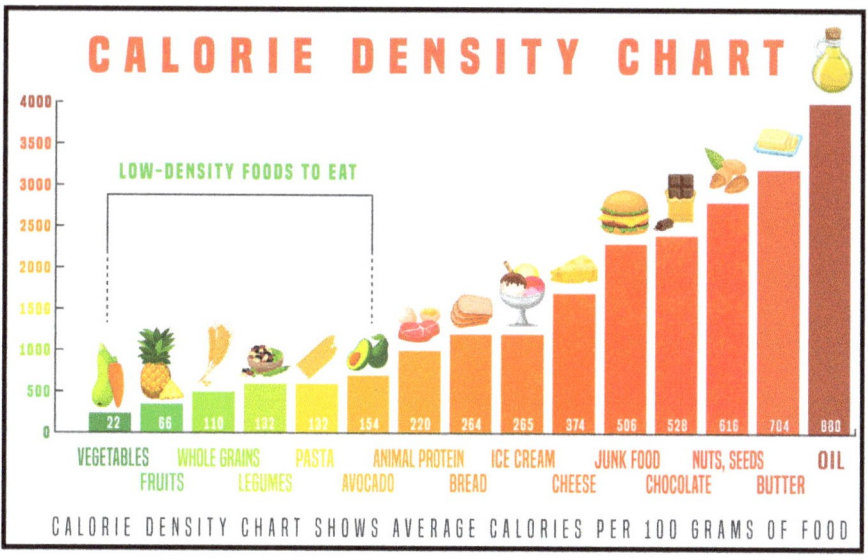

Caroline

Claire pops back into the room after putting her clothes in the dryer. "What about exercising before you eat? Does that burn fat?"

Jada shakes her head. "If you exercise without eating, muscles don't contract as well, and they use less energy, causing the workout to be less intense. So, after a cardio workout, your body burns less fat than usual, and you don't see as much gain in strength after resistance training, either.

"Meal timing is really important—eat when your body needs fuel, including when you wake up, and before and after exercise."

"That's actually simple," Claire says.

"The morning meal sets the tone, and then we can eat less in the afternoon and evening if we have any weight to lose. A calorie deficit at the end of the day, when the body doesn't need the fuel, won't disrupt our hormones."

"No fuel, no exercise," Caroline states, as if stamping a reminder in her brain.

"You got it. And stop eating a few hours before you go to bed so your body can focus on repair and recovery, not digestion."

The following week, Jada visits her brother and nieces, who are in town for a swim meet. She hears the girls talking about a teammate who missed her last few periods.

"She's not as fast as she was last year. Her times have gone up in all her events—freestyle, backstroke, and butterfly. Coach says losing your period is a symptom of under-fueling, and without enough nutrition, you can't maintain strength and speed," Jackie explains to her aunt.

Jada quietly connects the dots. A calorie deficit, or under-fueling, causes a breakdown of muscle tissue as the body uses its own resources for energy. It makes sense, considering what she recently learned about fasting.

During the reproductive years, missing a period is a very observable clue that the body is trying to protect itself while focusing on survival. There's no reason to put energy into creating a new life if resources are scarce.

After the reproductive years, signs of under-fueling become less obvious, but recognizing them is still essential. An energy deficiency can disrupt thyroid function and bone formation in as little as four days and eventually impact all the systems in the body.

Claire calls Jada. "How much protein do I need?"

Jada puts an earbud in and continues her walk. "It's complicated."

"I've got time if you do." Claire is stuck in rush-hour traffic and happy Jada answered.

"First, remember what our body does with protein. It breaks it down into amino acids, which are the building blocks for repairing tissue, making enzymes and antibodies, and maintaining muscle.

"So, the current Recommended Dietary Allowance (RDA) for protein is 0.36 grams per pound of body weight per day for healthy adults. A woman weighing 150 pounds requires 150 x 0.36 = 54 grams of protein per day. How much protein do you eat?" Jada asks.

"No clue," Claire responds.

"Well, the average adult female in the U.S. consumes 69 grams of protein per day. But I can show you an app where you can track for a few days and figure out *your* daily average."

Jada continues. "The guidelines for athletes who are strength training or doing endurance sports vary by organization, but some recommend as much as 0.9 grams per pound of body weight per day. This would increase the target for a 150-lb woman to 135 grams of protein each day."

Claire interjects, "That's way more than the RDA."

"I like to think in terms of percentages for the macronutrients—protein, carbs, and fat. If a woman consumes 2,000 calories per day and 540 of those calories are from protein (135 grams x 4 calories/gram = 540 calories), we can target about 25% of calories coming from protein. Does that make sense?"

Claire has trouble following the numbers while driving. "I'll have to go over this with you in person. In the meantime, send me the app, and I'll see if I can figure out how to track my protein for the rest of the week."

"Also," Jada adds, "consider the source of protein. There are benefits to consuming plant proteins over animal proteins. All whole plant foods contain protein, but you could focus on legumes and seeds for the biggest impact."

"Got it. Thanks."

PERCENT OF CALORIES FROM PROTEIN

Legumes

Lentils: ~31%
Edamame: ~38%
Chickpeas: ~31%
Black beans: ~31%
Split peas: ~30%

Soy-based Foods

Tofu: ~40%
Tempeh: ~40%
Soy milk: ~30%

Seeds

Hemp seeds: ~33%
Pumpkin seeds: ~33%
Flaxseeds: ~30%

Claire parks outside the grocery store. "What about carbs?"

"Carbs are great for energy. But just like protein, be thoughtful of the *type* of carbohydrate."

"What do you mean?" Claire asks.

Jada explains, "Simple carbs, like fruit, and complex carbs, like oats, beans, and potatoes, promote good health by supplying fuel to our cells for all our activities.

"Highly processed carbs, like sugary cereals, chips, and soda, can be harmful and are linked to many chronic diseases like obesity, diabetes, heart disease, and cancer. Focus on whole plant foods for the right type of carbohydrates, which include fiber to feed your gut bacteria."

"What about fats? Are they bad except for omega-3s?"

"Omega-3s are one type of unsaturated fat, but the other fats from plant foods are beneficial for health, too. The best sources are nuts, seeds, avocados, edamame, and other soy-based foods."

Jada adds, "Remember, fat is the most calorically dense of the macros. A good starting point in the diet is 25 to 30 percent of calories from fat. Lowering the percentage of fat may help when trying to lose weight and change body composition."

OVERNIGHT OATS WITH APPLES AND CINNAMON

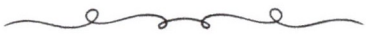

SERVES: 1   PREP TIME: 5 MINUTES

INGREDIENTS:

½ cup rolled oats
½ cup unsweetened soymilk (adjust for creaminess)
1 small apple, diced (keep the peel for extra fiber)
1 teaspoon ground cinnamon
1 teaspoon maple syrup (optional, for sweetness)
1 tablespoon chia seeds (optional, for thickness)
1 tablespoon chopped walnuts or almonds (optional)

DIRECTIONS:

Combine Ingredients: In a jar or bowl, mix the oats, soymilk, chia seeds (if using), and cinnamon. Stir well to combine.
Add the Apple: Stir in the diced apple. If you like a sweeter flavor, add the maple syrup.
Seal and Refrigerate: Cover the jar or bowl and refrigerate overnight (or at least 6 hours).
Serve: In the morning, give the oats a good stir. Add a splash of extra soymilk if they seem too thick. Top with walnuts or almonds for crunch, if desired.
Enjoy: Eat chilled or warm it up in the microwave for 1–2 minutes if you prefer it warm.

TIP:

Prepare 5 jars at the same time and have them ready all week!

EASY OATMEAL BREAKFAST COOKIES

PREP TIME: 15 MINUTES   MAKES: 8-12 COOKIES

INGREDIENTS:

1 large mashed banana
1/2 cup almond butter
1/4 cup maple syrup
2 teaspoons vanilla extract
1 cup old fashioned oats
1/4 cup whole wheat flour
1/4 cup ground flax seed
2 teaspoons ground cinnamon
1/2 teaspoon baking soda
1/4 cup raisins
1/4 cup chocolate chips

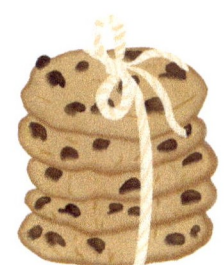

DIRECTIONS:

Prep: Preheat oven to 350 F.
Line cookie sheet with parchment paper; set aside.
Stir the First 4 Ingredients: In a large bowl, stir together banana, almond butter, maple syrup, and vanilla. (An immersion blender is handy for this step.)
Add the Solids: Add the oats, flour, ground flax, cinnamon, and baking soda and stir into the banana mixture until combined. Stir in raisins and chocolate chips.
Turn Batter into Cookies: Drop mounds of dough 3 inches apart on prepared cookie sheets. Makes 8-12 cookies. Bake for 14 to 16 minutes or until browned.
For maximal freshness, store in the fridge or the freezer.

My fave!

4
MUSCLES AFTER MENOPAUSE
Strength Training

Serena is sitting in the staff lounge, waiting for her lunch to heat up. She wraps her fingers around the back of her upper arm and squeezes the flesh between her thumb and index finger. "I'm getting too bulky. Maybe I should cut back on strength training."

Gail, Serena's co-worker, is perched on a stool at the counter. "Maybe you're not doing the right type of strength training. Do you think that's all muscle?" Gail asks in her typical unfiltered but nonjudgmental way while pointing to Serena's tricep area.

"What else would it be?" Serena asks.

"It could be fat. Are you in your forties yet?" Gail wonders.

"Yeah, I'm forty-six."

"Women's hormone levels change as we get older, and we're prone to losing muscle mass and storing fat. And we even store fat *in* the muscles, so instead of just solid muscle fibers, there's marbling from the fatty infiltration." Gail searches for an image of marbling in a muscle and shows it to Serena.

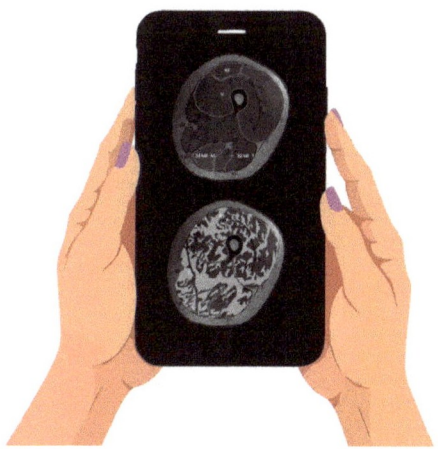

"Why does that happen?" Serena adjusts the tight sleeves on her scrub top.

"As women reach menopause and estrogen levels decrease, it's harder to stimulate muscle growth. Strength and power are the first to go, and then muscle mass starts to disappear."

3 Components of Muscle

Muscle mass: the physical size of the muscles
Strength: the ability of muscles to generate force
Power: the ability to exert force quickly

"But," Gail throws her hand in the air to emphasize the point, "we can slow the decline in muscle mass and muscle quality by increasing the resistance when we work out."

"How much resistance do we need?" Serena sounds anxious. She doesn't want to lose muscle mass, but she doesn't want to get injured either.

"Pick a weight heavy enough that you can only perform five reps with excellent form without being totally fatigued. It should feel like you could do two more if you had to, but you don't really want to. Those are called 'reps-in-reserve.'

"Then, rest for a few minutes and do five reps again. Work your way up to a total of five sets." Gail holds up her hand with her fingers outstretched.

"I do two sets of twelve to fifteen reps. It's really the same total work. Why would changing the number of reps and sets make a difference?" Serena looks confused.

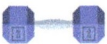

Old way: 2 sets x 12–15 reps = 24–30 reps

New way: 5 sets x 5 reps = 25 reps

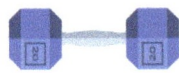

"Muscular fatigue in fewer reps is associated with the creation of power and strength—the qualities of our muscle that were supported by estrogen," Gail explains.

"Once we stop making estrogen, this type of heavy training—lower reps with more resistance—fills in the gap because it stimulates the central nervous system. And your brain responds with faster nerve signaling and stronger contractions. Does that make sense?"

"I think so. You're saying estrogen used to help with strength and power, and now that it's gone, I need to be more aggressive and create a CNS (central nervous system) response to preserve muscle?"

"Exactly. You're using the nervous system response—instead of estrogen—to stimulate the muscles." Gail pretends to do a challenging goblet squat with an imaginary dumbbell.

Serena wonders, "Can we just take HRT to increase estrogen and continue with the usual workout?"

"Hormone replacement therapy might reduce some of the unwanted symptoms of menopause, but it's not recreating the same hormonal environment you had during your reproductive years. You can't just add estrogen and expect the body to respond the same way. Instead, you need to find new ways to stimulate muscle cells."

Gail realizes she and Serena are on the same shift, and they will both get off at three today. "If you're going to the gym after work today, we could lift together."

"That would be amazing! I really appreciate it. I'll see you there." Serena rinses her lunch dishes, repacks her tote, and heads back to the floor to see patients.

Several hours later, Serena is in the gym looking for Gail who bounds in with a smile on her face. Gail explains the plan, which starts with a warm-up, including jumping exercises to build bone strength, followed by two upper-body exercises.

5x5: Complete all sets of the first exercise before moving to the second one.

EXERCISE	SET 1		SET 2		SET 3		SET 4		SET 5	
	WEIGHT	REPS	WEIGHT	REPS	WEIGHT	REPS	WEIGHT	REPS	WEIGHT	REPS
Chest Press										
Single Arm Row										

"Let's do chest presses and rows." Gail walks toward the dumbbell rack. With a quick hip bump, she maneuvers past her good friend Phil, the phlebotomist, as he tries to block her path.

Gail grabs a set of dumbbells, points to a pair for Serena, and walks over to one of the benches. "We can share the bench and do straight sets. I'll do five reps, and then I'll rest while you do five."

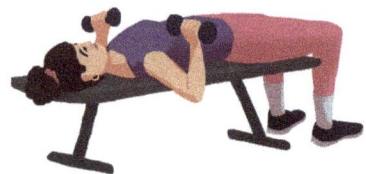

After five sets of chest presses, they complete five rounds of dumbbell rows.

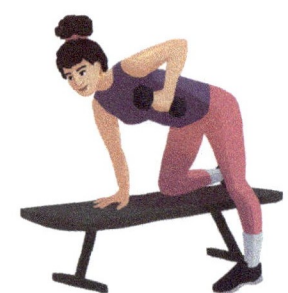

"Do you have time for a few other exercises—tricep extensions and bicep curls?"

Optional Upper Body Strength Exercises:
Alternate exercises with minimal rest for 10-12 reps.

EXERCISE	SET 1		SET 2		SET 3	
	WEIGHT	REPS	WEIGHT	REPS	WEIGHT	REPS
Bicep Curls						
Tricep Extensions						

"Let's do it."

After three sets of upper arm exercises, Serena picks up her phone and water bottle. "That was great. I like the 5x5 format and the superset at the end."

"Do you want to meet up tomorrow and work lower body?" Gail asks.

"Absolutely. It's fun to try something new. And if it works, I'll be even happier!" Serena grabs her keys and heads for the parking garage, ready to research the relationship between muscle and estrogen when she gets home.

The next day, Gail and Serena meet after work to do lower body exercises. Gail mentions next week's schedule change. "I picked up Dante's shift on Monday so instead of splitting our workouts, would you have time to do both upper and lower body on Tuesday?"

"Sure. What's your usual workout routine for the week?" Serena asks.

"Typically, Monday and Thursday are upper body, and Tuesday and Friday are lower body. Wednesday is a recovery day. On weekends, I try to get outside to hike or bike.

"When I pick up shifts, I'll do a longer full-body session to combine two days."

Gail elaborates, "When I was in my thirties, I did three total body workouts each week with at least one day of rest in between. But it takes me a little longer to recover now, so I changed to the split routine where I focus on upper body one day and lower body the next. Having two full days to rest the muscles between sessions feels better for my body."

"And we know the recovery is where the magic happens." Serena pulls her hair back into a ponytail, ready to get started.

Gail and Serena warm up with bodyweight squats and glute bridges to prepare for goblet squats and hip thrusts.

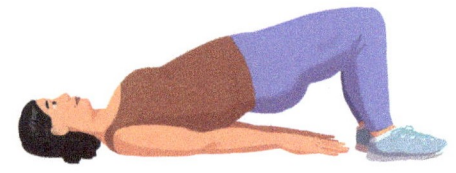

EXERCISE	Set 1		Set 2		Set 3		Set 4		Set 5	
	WEIGHT	REPS	WEIGHT	REPS	WEIGHT	REPS	WEIGHT	REPS	WEIGHT	REPS
Goblet Squat	25	5	30	5	30	5	30	4	25	5
Hip Thrust										

After they finish goblet squats and get ready for hip thrusts, Serena says, "I told my sister about our lifting routine. Sounds like she might try it."

"That's great. Has she done any strength training before?" Gail asks.

"I don't think so. She's always played tennis, but I don't think she lifts weights."

"Make sure she finds someone to help her with the movement patterns so she learns proper form. Taking time to build a good foundation, even if it's six months or a year, will pay off, and then she can start to add weight." Gail grabs two dumbbells to put on her hips and lies down on a mat with her knees bent and feet flat on the floor.

"Good point. I'll make sure she understands we are training for life, so there's no need to rush into it.

"She seemed reluctant about the jumping we did in the warmup for bone strength because her bladder leaks." Serena and Gail complete five reps of hip thrusts and set the dumbbells back down.

"Has she seen anyone about strengthening her pelvic floor muscles? Bladder issues are common in women, especially as we get older, and it's good to start those specific exercises sooner rather than later."

"I've told her to do Kegels, but I'll encourage her to see a specialist." Serena does ten repetitions every morning when her alarm goes off, squeezing the muscles that stop urination for a few seconds, then releasing and repeating.

Where did Gail get her Fitness Journal?

The fitness journal that accompanies this book is designed for women who are comfortable with strength training. If you have little or no experience, please seek appropriate guidance because proper form is crucial to prevent injury.

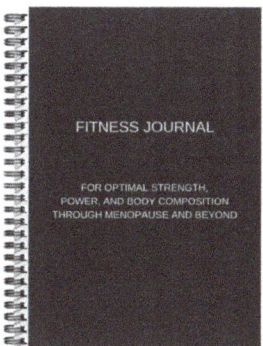

12 Week Fitness Journal

Start with five basic movements that are the foundation for every other movement—hinge, squat, push, pull, and single leg movements. Always emphasize quality over quantity. Make sure quality of movement is considered before volume and load.

5
HOLLOW BONES ARE FOR HUMMINGBIRDS

Bone Health

Anika worries about her bones. Last week, she had her first DEXA scan to evaluate her bone density. Her mother, Anabel, is frail and was diagnosed with osteoporosis decades ago.

"I don't understand," Anika wails, "I take calcium supplements and eat dairy every day!" She chews dramatically on a cheese stick and sips on her latte.

"What happened?" Valerie sits on the sofa with her legs up on the chaise.

"My doctor called and said my T score is low. I have osteopenia."

"Is that the stage before osteoporosis?" Xia is perched cross-legged in the chair on the other side of the coffee table with a book in her lap.

"Yup, that's how it starts. The scan shows my bone density is lower than it should be." Anika's voice fills with fear.

Evaluating Bone Density

What is a DEXA Scan?

A DEXA (Dual-Energy X-Ray Absorptiometry) scan is a quick, non-invasive imaging test that measures bone density. The test is used to diagnose osteoporosis and assess fracture risk.

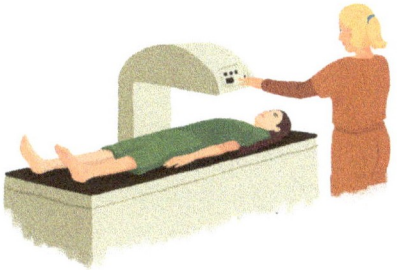

What is a T-Score?

The **T-score** compares a woman's result to the average peak bone density of a healthy thirty-year-old woman.

BONE MINERAL DENSITY: T Scores

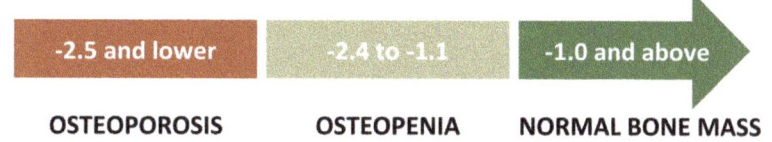

-2.5 and lower	-2.4 to -1.1	-1.0 and above
OSTEOPOROSIS	OSTEOPENIA	NORMAL BONE MASS

"Okay, deep breath. Bone density is only one marker of bone strength. The other is bone quality," Valerie explains.

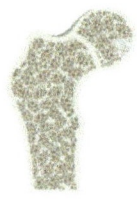 **Bone strength is a combination of both *density* and *quality*.**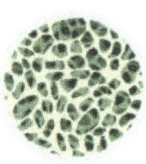

"What's the difference between bone density and bone quality?" Xia asks.

"Bone density refers to the amount of minerals, like calcium and phosphorus, in the bone. That's what the DEXA scan measures. But, you can also use another test called the trabecular bone score, or TBS, to determine the quality of the bone.

"The TBS uses the data from the DEXA scan to evaluate the spongy part of the bone that looks like a honeycomb. This helps create a more accurate assessment of overall bone strength."

Valerie adds, "But not all DEXA scanners include the TBS software, so you need to look for specific locations to have it done."

"Does good bone quality lessen the likelihood of breaking a bone?" Anika says hopefully.

"Totally. And on the flip side, sometimes you see poor bone quality even when the T-score is normal. In those cases, they will be at a greater risk of fracture."

"Why would that happen?" Xia and Anika say at the same time.

"Diseases like diabetes and rheumatoid arthritis can weaken the bone architecture without the bone mineral density dropping below normal," Valerie explains.

"I didn't know diabetes can weaken bones!" Xia thinks of her brother, who has been living with the disease for many years.

"The bone matrix gets weak from the effects of high blood sugar and inflammation. The normal bone turnover—getting rid of old bone and laying down new bone—gets disrupted. Just another reason to be vigilant about diabetes treatment." Valerie takes a sip from her coffee cup.

"So if the T score is low, but the TBS is high, there's less to worry about?" Anika plans to ask her doctor about this test.

"That will likely make the fracture risk lower, but the point is there's a lot to consider besides the T score. Just be sure to get the full picture so you can understand your specific situation."

Valerie continues, "There are ways to actively improve bone health. If your doctor says it's safe, you can do jump training to increase bone density. The pressure on the bones can stimulate them the same way lifting weights strengthens muscles.

"And actually, lifting weights strengthens bones too. The tendons at the ends of the muscles attach to the bones. They pull on the bones, and that's another signal for bone growth."

"Do jumping jacks count?" Xia asks.

"Absolutely. And skipping or playing hopscotch."

"Do I need to do it every day?" Anika stresses about time.

"A few times a week can improve bone density, but talk to your doctor first. Let's discuss more tonight. I'm taking Vince for his driver's test."

"Fingers crossed!" her friends shout after her.

Benefits of Jump Training

Jumping not only builds bone, but it also helps build power in the muscles.

Power accelerates control and coordination of muscle movements and helps the body recover in situations where a fall could occur.

Start with something small like bodyweight jump squats and work your way up to hopping off a low step.

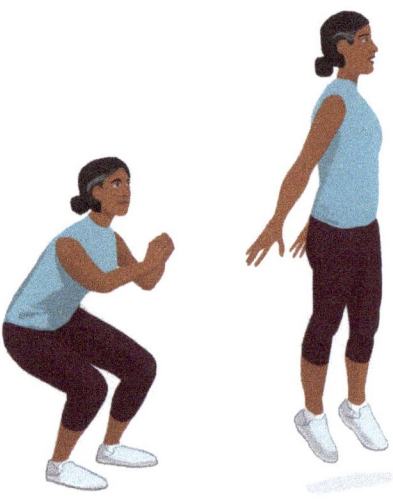

"Are you kidding me? There are estrogen receptors in our bones?" Anika asks Valerie as they volley to warm up for Thursday night pickleball with their husbands, Andre and Victor.

"It's true. Estrogen plays an important role in bone density. Low estrogen levels during menopause accelerate bone loss, which is why so many women develop osteoporosis after the transition." Valerie bends down to tie her shoe.

"What does estrogen do to bone?"

"It encourages the formation of new bone. Without estrogen, bones can lose density and become brittle.

"Every minute of every day, bones are breaking down and rebuilding. The turnover helps maintain the strength of our skeleton. Specific cells break down the old, damaged bone, and other cells build new bone.

"Think of the construction on the beltway. At any given time, a section of the highway is being torn up by one piece of equipment and repaved by another. If the repaving didn't occur, the road would get weaker with more potholes and start to fall apart."

"Estrogen helps with the repaving?" Anika imagines fresh asphalt filling in holes.

"It does. It also taps the brakes on the equipment tearing up the road to keep the whole process well-balanced."

"Are we doomed after menopause?" Anika lunges for a ball coming to her left.

"No, we aren't doomed. Women live active lives into their 80s and 90s even when their bone density is lower than average. You just need to keep your bones and muscles as strong as possible."

"By jumping and strength training?" Anika asks.

"You got it. But you need to use enough resistance—whether it's with dumbbells, cables, or bands—to cause the muscles to pull on the bones. A study called LiftMOR (I love that name) took a hundred women with low bone density and split them into two groups—high-intensity and low-intensity lifting. Both groups worked out twice a week for thirty minutes. After eight months, the heavy lifters significantly improved the bone density in their hips and spines."

"Calcium from milk is important too, right?" Anika remembers the big push in her youth to drink milk, *It does a body good.*

"Actually, in countries consuming the most milk, fracture rates are not lower than in countries where people consume less dairy. The U.S. has one of the highest rates of milk consumption on the planet and one of the highest rates of hip fractures!"

Anika stops and walks to the net to get water. "What?"

"Yeah, it's crazy. When we're talking about nutrition and bone health, calcium is just the tip of the iceberg. A well-balanced diet filled with unprocessed food is the best way to eat. Our bodies know how to break down whole foods to get the nutrients we need like phosphorus and magnesium which are also important for building bone." Valerie takes a sip from her water bottle.

"I'm so shocked by the milk and fracture rates." Anika shakes her head.

"I know, right? In one of the biggest studies, researchers looked at the diets of 77,000 nurses over twelve years and found that women who drank two or more glasses of milk per day, or consumed more calcium from food, did not have a lower risk of hip fracture than women who drank milk just once a week."

"It's hard to fathom that consuming more milk doesn't lower the risk of fractures," Anika says. "What about Vitamin D?"

"It's definitely important because the body can't absorb calcium without it. Vitamin D isn't found in many foods, but we can make it when our skin is exposed to sunlight. Have you ever had your Vitamin D level checked?"

"I'm pretty sure my doctor checks it at my annual exam in the spring. She says it's a good time of year to check Vitamin D since we have the least amount of sun exposure in the winter." Anika looks at her bare, pale arms.

"Right. That would give you a sense of its lowest level during the year," Valerie explains.

"Is there anything I should avoid to keep my bones healthy?" Anika asks.

"Sure, but you already avoid soda and alcohol, which rob bones of minerals." Valerie knows Anika drinks water every day and orders mocktails when they're out. "You could focus on eating anti-inflammatory foods like fruits and vegetables and minimizing sugar and refined carbs to keep inflammation low."

"What if I eat right and exercise, but my T score doesn't improve?" Anika wonders about other options.

"Estrogen may help, especially since you are perimenopausal. The most rapid bone loss happens in the first five to eight years as estrogen starts to disappear," Valerie says.

"Refresh my memory. Why does that happen?"

"When estrogen isn't around, the osteoclasts—the cells breaking down bone—act like kids whose parents left town. They go wild at first, but eventually they slow down, and women lose bone at the same rate as men after that."

"So, hormones can help?" Anika wonders if she should ask her gynecologist about taking estrogen.

"Yup. They can reduce bone loss, increase bone density, and reduce the risk of fracture. But be aware, the benefits only last as long as you take the medication."

"Does the form of estrogen matter?" Anika asks.

"Oral medications and skin patches are used in those cases, but vaginal creams won't work. They just stay in the local tissue and don't reach the bloodstream."

Andre and Victor stroll onto the court, and the two couples begin the game. In the third game, Valerie trips over a ball left on the court from the previous point. She stumbles but regains her balance.

"Wow, nice recovery!" Anika shouts as she hurries over to pick up the loose ball.

"That reminds me—balance exercises! I can't believe I forgot to mention earlier that the best way to prevent a fracture is not to fall!

"I'll text you later with some balance exercises to try. I do them for about five minutes every day when I'm on the phone or watching TV."

"Sounds great—thanks!"

Valerie

Here are the balance exercises.

For each exercise, be sure to stand up straight and engage your core.

1. Single-leg stand: 10-30 seconds per side.
2. Heel-to-toe walk: heel of one foot touches toes of the other, 20 steps.
3. Side leg lifts: lift leg out to the side and lower it, 10-15 reps per side.
4. Tree Pose: stand on one leg, rest other foot on calf. 10-30 seconds per side.

Anika

What's a heel-to-toe walk?

Valerie

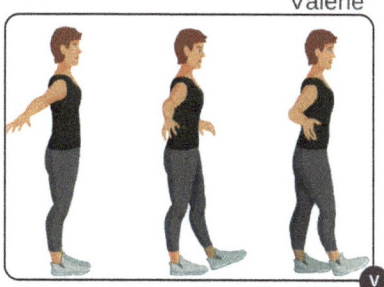

6
TO SIT OR NOT TO SIT

Maximal Efforts

Paula and Lori arrive at the gym for their workout with a new trainer, Tracy.

Their usual trainer, Ted, is on paternity leave. His wife went into labor during their last session.

"Her water broke!" he shouted after pulling his vibrating phone out of his pocket. Paula and Lori smile, remembering the excitement of having their own firstborn, and hurry Ted out of the gym to meet his wife at the hospital.

Tracy greets the women with a fist bump and starts the session with inchworms to loosen up. The ladies hinge at the hips and walk their hands out past a pushup position.

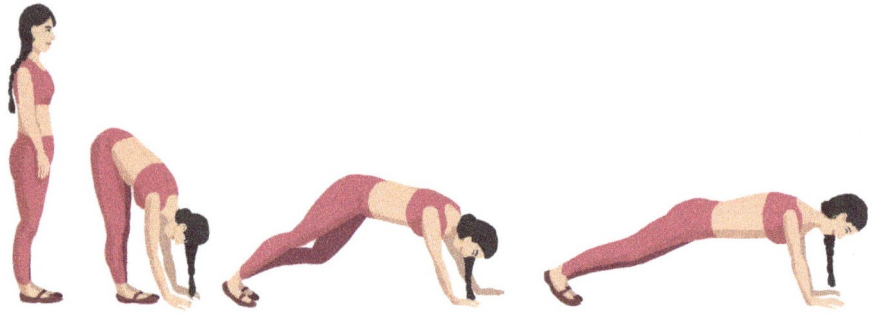

Paula exclaims, "I really hate these! It may sound ridiculous, but I can just feel my belly hanging down, and it's freakin' annoying!"

Tracy hears the frustration in Paula's voice and sees Lori nodding in agreement. "Let's talk for a minute before we get started today. I'll be with you for the next six weeks. I may do things a little differently from Ted, and I want to be sure we're on the same page."

The three women sit on a mat in the stretching area. Paula and Lori answer Tracy's questions about family, lifestyle, and goals. "So, your top three issues are fatigue, trouble sleeping, and weight gain." Tracy looks for confirmation from Paula and Lori.

Paula replies, "I think if I could sleep well, everything else would fall into place."

"It could be an imbalance in your hormones. You probably know about the changes in estrogen and progesterone levels as we women age. Did you know those changes cause a lot of stress on the body internally? And when the body is stressed, cortisol gets released. We end up with a new elevated baseline for cortisol, which causes a weird state of 'tired but wired.'"

"I guess that's why I feel exhausted but can't sleep," Lori realizes.

Tracy continues, "And it's all connected. High cortisol levels contribute to poor sleep. Fatigue disrupts our hunger cues. And, the elevated cortisol not only increases cravings but also promotes fat storage. For many women, weight gain seems inevitable."

Lori wonders if there is any way to turn this around. "Can we bring the cortisol down?"

Tracy smiles. "Yes! If we exercise at a higher intensity, we can stimulate the release of other hormones that will lower our cortisol. In order to be effective, the work is short in duration but demanding in effort.

"HIIT, high-intensity interval training, or SIT, sprint interval training, are both good ways to increase the intensity of your workout, and you really only need to do it two or three times a week."

Paula smiles. "I know about HIIT—twenty seconds of work, ten seconds of rest, for eight rounds. It was developed by a Japanese speed skating coach, right?"

Tracy nods. "I'm impressed. Tabata is one of the most well-known protocols, but you can adjust the time intervals and number of rounds for HIIT. The idea is to have short bursts of effort with even shorter recoveries until your efforts lose their intensity."

Lori asks, "What is SIT?"

Tracy explains, "SIT is a type of HIIT—it's an all-out max effort for ten to thirty seconds followed by a few minutes of recovery. You start with one or two rounds and work up to more. If you can ever go above seven or eight rounds, you're probably not going as hard as you need to."

"That sounds tough." Paula looks nervous.

"Remember, it's only thirty seconds at most. And just imagine the muscle and bone stimulation happening during the exercise, not to mention the metabolic changes.

"During these bursts, glucose uptake in the muscles improves, and the ability to burn fat increases. And the high intensity lowers blood pressure by dilating the blood vessels in an effort to send more blood and oxygen to the muscles."

Tracy asks, "So, do you want to do HIIT or SIT today?"

"I'll definitely SIT!" Lori jokes, striking a chair pose from her mental yoga library.

"All right. Remember, SIT stands for Sprint Interval Training, so we'll go hard, but for a short time. The intervals will fire up your fast-twitch muscle fibers, not the slow-twitch you use for endurance. We'll start with one or two intervals per session, and we only do these two or three times a week. You don't need more."

Lori strides over to the treadmill. "Who goes first?"

"Sprinting doesn't mean you need to run. You can do lots of activities at max effort. You could bike or row if you don't want to sprint on the treadmill," Tracy explains.

In postmenopausal women, some research suggests cycling is better than running for high-intensity training. It may be easier to hit the higher intensities on the bike with less pressure on the joints.

"I'll bike," Paula chimes in. "But give me a few minutes; I'll be right back."

As Paula heads to the locker room, Lori turns to Tracy. "How padded are the bike seats? I tried to ride last summer with my family in Yellowstone, and it was too painful."

Tracy sympathizes, "If the seat isn't comfortable, you can wear padded bike shorts or try a medicated cream to address the issue more directly. Once women go through menopause, the vaginal tissues get dry and brittle, and as you probably know, this affects way more than the ability to ride a bike!"

Lori nods her head. "No doubt about that. Where do I get the cream?"

To Sit or Not to Sit

"Talk to your gynecologist. They have an estrogen cream that stays localized to the vaginal tissue, so it doesn't carry any of the risks of hormone replacement."

Tracy guides Lori and Paula through a ten-minute warmup routine, including bodyweight squats and inverted flyers.

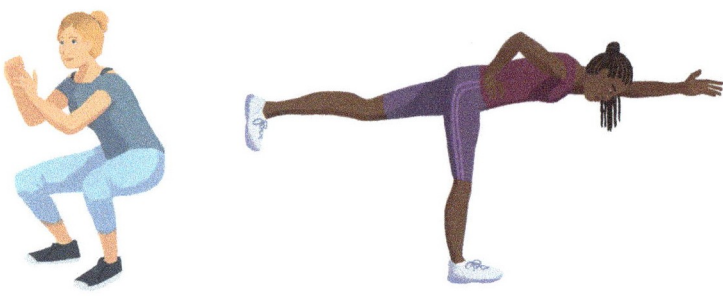

"Okay. Paula, adjust your bike, and Lori, start the treadmill, but don't hop on yet. I'll tell you when to start. We'll go for twenty seconds.

Lori and Paula get ready, and on Tracy's signal, Lori sprints and Paula pedals. Tracy notices Paula's legs are slowing down after fifteen seconds. The timer goes off, and the ladies are audibly grateful.

Tracy discusses the strategy for the second round. "This time will be fifteen seconds," she says.

"I can do twenty!" Paula replies adamantly.

"I know, but I don't want you to lose good form or subconsciously slow down to make it to the end of the twenty seconds. That defeats the purpose. Remember, it's not about how long you can work; it's about working at maximum effort to cause the release of hormones that lower cortisol."

"Oh, I get it."

"Quality over quantity," Lori adds.

After a 3-minute rest, Paula and Lori start the second round. They push at max effort for fifteen seconds and understand why Tracy adjusted the time.

> ### Will HIIT increase our cortisol levels?
>
> It will, but that is not a bad thing. During high intensity training, we create acute stress in the body. Cortisol levels spike to cause the release of adrenaline which increases heart rate and oxygen consumption. This is very different from the long-term effects of chronic cortisol elevation.

"I think I was at max effort the whole time!" Lori says breathlessly.

"Me too! And that helps reset our baseline cortisol level?" Paula asks.

"Yes. This sudden spike in cortisol stimulates the release of growth hormone and testosterone, which will lower cortisol levels, promote the repair of tissues, and create new muscle," Tracy explains. "But you need to hit that high intensity to get the results.

After two rounds of the SIT workout, the women return to the mat for mobility, balance, and core training.

"I don't feel like I've done enough work today," Paula worries.

Tracy nods. "In the past, training programs were written for long, grueling sessions. With more research available, we realize more is not always better. Continuous training keeps stress on the body and does not allow cortisol to return to its lower levels. It's about working smarter."

"My sister goes to the new fitness place in town, and she says they do interval training. The classes are at least forty-five minutes, if not an hour. Is that HIIT?" Lori asks.

"It's hard to say. It could be, but in group classes, it's not easy to push to maximum effort when you're following an instructor or surrounded by people mimicking each other's movements."

Paula rolls her calves on the foam roller. "So, if we do HIIT or SIT two or three times a week, what else should we be doing? I mean, that workout didn't take long. Should I get on the elliptical or treadmill for another half hour?"

No. The continuous stress will keep cortisol elevated. You should give your body time to relax and recover.

"You have a dog, right?" Tracy remembers from their earlier conversation that Lori and Paula both rescued dogs recently.

"I have a rescue from last year's hurricane in Florida. She's so adorable!" Paula holds up her phone and shares a picture.

"Take her for a walk. You'll keep your blood flowing, which helps with recovery, but you won't be adding more stress.

"Think of this new way of training like a light switch—it's either ON with focused effort or OFF with recovery. If you try to use a dimmer, you won't create the change you need to get the results you want.

"Using RPE—rating of perceived exertion—is a good way to gauge intensity. Interval training should be at an eight or above on a scale of one to ten."

RPE: RATING OF PERCEIVED EXERTION SCALE

How hard are you working on a scale of 1-10?
Low Intensity = 1 to 3
Moderate Intensity = 4 to 7
High Intensity = 8 to 10

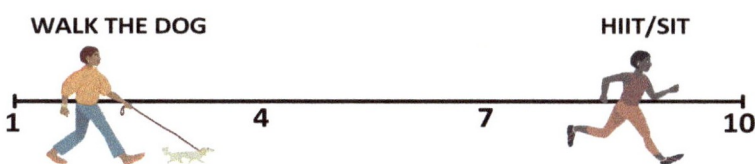

Lori mentions, "I recently read an article recommending 150 minutes of moderate-intensity exercise each week."

Tracy replies, "If a woman doesn't have a fitness routine, that's probably a good idea. It would at least take her from inactive to active. But for women who have been putting forth an effort and not getting the results they want, it's time to look at newer research. Most exercise guidelines are based on studies using men. More recent research focuses on women's unique physiology and allows us to be smarter about our training.

"The combination of low estrogen and high cortisol changes our body composition—we lose muscle and gain fat—so we need to alter our workouts to deal with the new hormonal situation."

"I would think doing more cardio would burn more fat." Lori is struggling with this new way of thinking.

"Prolonged cardio at a moderate intensity puts moderate stress on the body and releases more cortisol.

"There's a lot more to consider than just burning calories. We need to consider everything going on in the body to make real changes. Hormones dictate how calories are used or stored and are a critical factor in our exercise selection."

Lori and Paula smile. "So, what's the plan for tomorrow, coach?"

Tracy smiles. "Tomorrow is resistance training. Ted's plan shows weights on Tuesdays."

"Great!" the women say simultaneously. They leave the gym with a lot of new information to process and are eager to return and learn more from their new trainer.

HIGH INTENSITY CARDIO INTERVALS
RPE = Rating of Perceived Exertion
How hard are you working on a scale of 0-10?

SIT
Sprint Interval Training

RPE* 10
Work: 10-30 seconds
Recover: 2-3 minutes
Up to 8 rounds

HIIT
High Intensity Interval Training

RPE* 8-9
Work & Rest Intervals:
1-4 minutes
Recover: 1 minute
1-3 rounds

SIT Activities: Work 10-30 seconds at 100% effort.

Jump Squats	Treadmill Sprints
Battle Ropes	Fast Feet
Mountain Climbers	Jump Rope
Rower	Kettlebell Swings
Bike	Medicine Ball Slams

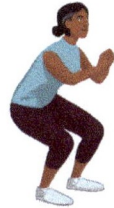  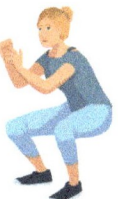

HIIT Activities: Work 1-4 minutes at 80% effort.

Tabata on bike:
20 seconds on / 10 seconds rest x 8 cycles = 4 minutes

EMOM (Every Minute On the Minute): Start the exercise at the top of each minute until you complete the number of repetitions, rest the remainder of that minute.

> Example:
> Minute 1: 15 thrusters, rest until 1:00
> Minute 2: 20 kettlebell swings, rest until 2:00
> Minute 3: 20 alternating reverse lunges, rest until 3:00
> Minute 4: 15 pushups, rest until 4:00.

7
FLEXIBLE FOR THE FUTURE

Tendons and Ligaments

Kim calls Emily on the way to work. "My left shoulder is still killing me. I can't figure out what's going on. I feel more and more limited in my activities, and the yard is getting out of control. The weeds are taking over!"

Emily, the wife of an orthopedic surgeon, sympathizes. "Yeah, I've been struggling with this plantar fasciitis, but I finally started physical therapy last week."

"Hey, do you think Ezra would mind taking a look at my shoulder when you drop the girls off after swim practice?" Kim reluctantly asks.

"I'm sure he won't mind. We'll be there around six." Emily hangs up and tells Ezra the plan.

"Thanks for the ride, Dr. and Mrs. Evans," Kirsten and Kathy say in unison as they jump out of the car.

"No problem, girls. We're coming in to talk to your mom."

Kim's discomfort is obvious as she greets everyone at the door.

Immediately, Ezra points to Kim's shoulder and asks, "When did this start?"

"I'm not sure. It's been getting worse over the past few weeks, but I can't think of a specific injury."

"Maybe there was a small event where you had a little tear but didn't notice at the time. With repeated use, it probably gets torn a little more each day. You have to give it more time to heal and lay off the yardwork."

"I know it's not fun to hear, but it takes longer to recover as we get older." Ezra glances from Kim to his wife. "And as estrogen levels decrease, there is less of the hormone around to stimulate collagen production. Tendons and ligaments get stiffer, and the healing process is slower."

Shoulder Instability

During and after the menopause transition, hormonal changes can cause the shoulder joint to become less stable. A decline in muscle mass and stiffer tendons around the rotator cuff can leave women vulnerable to shoulder injuries.

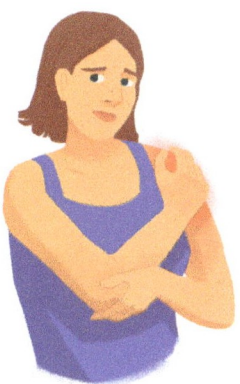

"I thought hormones make injuries more likely when we're young. Now you're telling me the loss of hormones during menopause makes us more injury-prone." Kim sighs.

"Remember last year when Kirsten tore her ACL in the soccer game? You and the trainer said it's more common in females after puberty because of estrogen binding to receptors on the ligament, making it looser." Hearing the familiar beep of the preheated oven, Kim turns and puts a lasagna on the middle shelf.

"Women definitely face challenges because of hormone changes," Ezra says. He motions toward the girls. "At that age, hormones affect the body by widening the hips, which changes the angle from the hip to the knee and puts the ligaments in a more vulnerable position.

"When the reproductive years end, tendons and ligaments get stiff because of a lack of estrogen. Stiff ligaments aren't as much of an issue. But stiff tendons cause more strain on the muscle and lead to tendon and muscle injuries. The most common issues involve the Achilles tendon and rotator cuff."

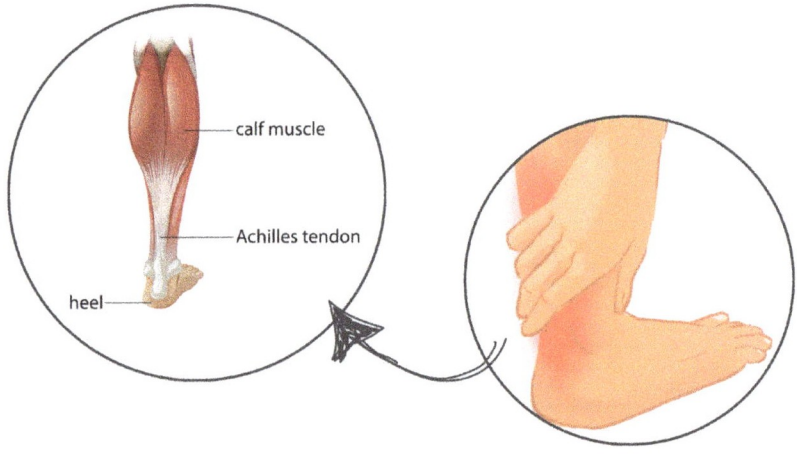

"What can I do?" Kim asks.

"Make time every day for soft tissue work—foam rolling or using a tennis or lacrosse ball to massage the muscles and tendons. Even just a few minutes will help keep them supple and increase blood flow to the area which helps repair any damage. Blood carries the nutrients cells need to recover.

"If you don't address the problem, it can become a cycle of injury, inflammation, scar tissue, and limited mobility; then another injury happens. Does that make sense?" Ezra takes a breath.

"It does, but foam rolling is *so* painful," Emily interjects.

"Pain confirms the tissues aren't healthy. But don't stay in the pain zone. Start with light pressure. It should feel slightly uncomfortable, but if you feel pain, back off. Or move to the area just above or below the point of tenderness like we did with your calves." Ezra says, pointing to his wife.

"What's wrong with your calves?" Kim inquires.

"Twenty years of wearing heels. It's like pointing your toes for two decades. And apparently it caused my Achilles to shorten." Emily huffs. Kim thinks about Emily's shoe closet, which is filled with the trendiest labels.

"Studies show the calf muscles in women who wore heels were thirteen percent shorter than calf muscles in women who wore flats," Ezra explains.

"High-heeled shoes cause other issues, too. Walking in heels keeps you from having a normal foot strike where you roll from heel to toe. Instead, all the pressure is on the toe and the front of the foot, causing the hip flexors to do the work. And then, tight hip flexors cause an exaggerated curve in the lower back and create muscle imbalances that can lead to injury.

"We should get out of your hair, but here's one more tip. Always warm up before any exercise, even yard work. And strength train and eat well." Ezra snatches an apple from the fruit bowl and tosses it in the air.

Kim smiles, thanks him, and sends her friends on their way.

KIM'S QUICK LASAGNA

SERVES: 4   PREP TIME: 35 MINUTES

INGREDIENTS:

16 ounces riced cauliflower, fresh or frozen
3 tablespoons lemon juice
2 tablespoons + 1/2 cup unsweetened nondairy milk
1 tablespoon + 1/4 cup nutritional yeast
1.5 teaspoons dried oregano
1 teaspoon salt
1/8 teaspoon black pepper
2 cups + 1 cup pasta or marinara sauce
6 ounces fresh baby spinach, finely chopped
1 box whole wheat lasagna

DIRECTIONS:

Preheat oven to 350 F.

Step One: Make the Cauliflower Ricotta
Start with riced cauliflower in a large mixing bowl.
Add lemon juice, nondairy milk (2T), nutritional yeast (1T), oregano, salt and pepper and mix well.

Step Two: Assemble the Lasagna
In a rectangular baking pan, layer the ingredients in this order: sauce, noodles, 1/2 of cauliflower ricotta, noodles, sauce, 1/2 of spinach, noodles, 1/2 of cauliflower ricotta, 1/2 of spinach, noodles.

For the top layer, mix the last 1 cup of sauce with 1/2 cup of nondairy milk and 1/4 cup nutritional yeast.
Pour over the top. Bake, uncovered, for 55 minutes (until noodles are cooked through).

8
SHOW ME THE SEROTONIN

Mood

Sage and Betsy stop at the luggage carousel after a short flight. They're attending a friend's wedding in New Orleans. Betsy grabs her bag and waits with Sage. As she gazes at the suitcases passing by, Sage feels tired and empty but hopes this weekend will rejuvenate her spirit.

Sage and Betsy decided to share a room and relive roommate days. "I started on an SSRI last year for anxiety and depression," Sage mumbles as she sets the prescription bottle on one side of the bathroom sink.

> ## SSRI = Selective Serotonin Reuptake Inhibitors
>
> **How do they work?** Increase serotonin levels in the brain
>
> **Examples:** Prozac, Zoloft, Paxil, Celexa

"Do you want to talk about it?" Betsy asks. "I'm sorry you're struggling."

"I don't know exactly why I feel depressed, but after talking to my doctor and a therapist, they recommended medication."

"Do you have menopause symptoms—like hot flashes, night sweats, or changes in your period?" Betsy asks.

"Yeah, my period is all over the place. Sometimes I bleed just a little, and other times, I can't leave the house. Why do you ask?"

"You might be perimenopausal," Betsy says, knowing she and Sage are the same age. The two women met at the health center when Betsy was starting her residency in obstetrics and gynecology, and Sage was a postdoctoral student in the research lab.

"Does perimenopause cause anxiety and depression?" Sage asks.

"Mental health changes can be a sign of shifting hormone levels. As menopause approaches, estrogen and progesterone levels dip and spike like a roller coaster winding down, with smaller, unpredictable hills that can throw your body for a loop.

"And that fluctuation wreaks havoc. Think about how moody teenagers are as hormone levels surge. Perimenopause brings a similar kind of turbulence—it's like hormone chaos, round two."

"Why did my doctor prescribe an SSRI and not HRT?" Sage asks.

"To increase serotonin. During premenopause—the years when we have regular periods—estrogen plays a role in serotonin production. But as estrogen levels decline, we make less serotonin, which can lead to depression along with hot flashes and night sweats. SSRIs are prescribed to help with any of these symptoms, especially for women who shouldn't take hormone therapy.

Betsy continues encouragingly, "But there are other ways we can help our bodies restore serotonin."

"Like what?" Sage desperately wants to feel better.

"Exercise is super helpful. Cardio and resistance training increase the release of serotonin in the brain. Do you exercise?" Betsy asks.

"A little. What else can I do?" Sage wants some less time-consuming options. And exercise seems daunting.

"Sunlight can help. Exposure to either the sun or a lightbox increases serotonin levels. People with the 'winter blues' have less serotonin, so light therapy is one of the main treatments for seasonal affective disorder."

"I can try to get outside more. Hera will love that." Sage smiles, thinking of her beautiful white German Shepherd who enjoys long walks on the old railroad trail.

"And one of the most important factors is food. One way to get more serotonin in your brain is to eat more vegetables, fruits, beans, nuts, seeds, and whole grains.

"Also, try to minimize foods high in fat, sugar, and salt. They're associated with anxiety and depression."

Sage asks, "Aren't nuts and seeds high in fat?"

"Yeah, but they have good fats, and they're healthy in small amounts. Think about how many you would eat if you had to take them out of the shell—probably a lot less than if you pour them from a bag. My advice would be to use them sparingly as a condiment."

"What do you mean?"

"You could sprinkle walnuts on oatmeal or pumpkin seeds on a salad," Betsy explains.

Betsy puts an arm around Sage. "How about we start with sun and exercise now, and then we'll find a nice spot for lunch?" The women leave the hotel and walk through City Park.

Two hours later, the women are rejuvenated by their conversation but famished from the walk. They see a restaurant that offers plant-based options and find a table. After ordering two Mediterranean Hummus Wraps, Sage asks, "What about probiotics? Do they help with mood?"

"Probiotics are simply bacteria. We have trillions of them in our gut, and maintaining the right balance of different strains is crucial for our health. But the composition of your gut bacteria is specific to you—like a fingerprint.

"So, it's better to feed the ones we have than to rely on bacteria from a pill. Adding supplemental probiotics can crowd out the natural bacteria and reduce its diversity," Betsy explains.

"You mean like last summer when mint took over my garden and choked out the basil and parsley?" Sage's mind wanders to her struggle with the herbs, and Betsy chuckles at the analogy.

"Totally, but eating whole plant foods and avoiding the highly processed stuff shifts your gut microbiome and results in higher quantities of good bacteria. The harmful bacteria die off, and you'll end up flushing those down the toilet."

"So, I have good *and* bad bacteria living in my gut?"

"Yes. Everyone has a unique microbiome, and the ratio of the different types of bacteria plays a huge role in both our physical and mental health. Unfortunately, starting around four or five years before menopause, changes in hormone levels can lead to a decrease in the diversity of our microbiome.

"This can mean fewer species of beneficial bacteria, which makes the gut less resilient. It affects how well nutrients get absorbed and how well the immune system responds to harmful bacteria.

"But it also means a reduction in our mood-boosting hormone. Ninety percent of serotonin is secreted by good bacteria in the gut. So, eating healthy plant foods to nourish them is essential."

"Wow—bacteria play a huge role in our health!" Sage is amazed at the impact of the microbiome.

Besty continues, "Bottom line—feed the good gut bacteria with whole plant foods."

"Why do I have to eat plants to feed them?" Sage asks.

"Because plants contain fiber, and that's what the bacteria eat. We digest our food in the small intestines, and it's only the fiber that makes it to the colon where most gut bacteria live."

"Okay." Sage repeats the information to make sure she understands, "Fruits, vegetables, whole grains, beans, nuts, and seeds. Got it. I'll focus on nutrition first, then think about adding more exercise. I can definitely get outside a few times each day to get some sun. Thanks for talking to me about this."

Trust Your Gut

Here are some good sources of fiber!

FRUITS

Raspberries – 8 g/cup
Pears (with skin) – 6 g*
Apples (with skin) – 4 g*

VEGETABLES

Brussels Sprouts – 4 g/cup**
Sweet Potatoes (with skin) – 4 g*
Spinach – 4 g/cup**
Cauliflower – 3 g/cup**
Zucchini (with skin) – 2 g/cup**
Artichokes – 10 g*
Broccoli – 5 g/cup**
Carrots – 4 g/cup raw

WHOLE GRAINS

Quinoa – 5 g/cup**
Oats – 4 g/cup**
Brown Rice – 3.5 g/cup**

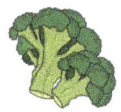

and a few more....

LEGUMES

Lentils – 16g/cup**
Black Beans – 15g/cup**
Chickpeas – 12.5g/cup**

NUTS

Walnuts – 2g/oz
(about 14 halves)
Almonds – 3.5g/oz
(about 23 nuts)
Pistachios – 3 g/oz
(about 49 nuts)

SEEDS

Pumpkin Seeds – 5g/oz
Sesame Seeds – 4g/oz
Chia Seeds – 10g/oz
Flaxseeds – 8g/oz

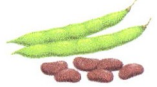
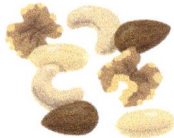

oz=ounce   g=grams   *medium size fruit or vegetable   **cooked

FIBER-FILLED FAJITAS

SERVES: 4   PREP TIME: 20 MINUTES

INGREDIENTS:

1 onion, diced
2 tablespoons garlic, minced
2 bell peppers, chopped (1 red, 1 green)
1 8-ounce pack of sliced mushrooms
1 tablespoon chili powder
1 teaspoon smoked paprika
1/2 teaspoon salt
1 can (15.5 ounces) black beans, drained and rinsed
1 can (15.5 ounces) pinto beans, drained and rinsed
Whole wheat or corn tortillas

DIRECTIONS:

Cook Vegetables: On a sheet pan in a 400 degree F oven, or using the stovetop, cook veggies until tender.

Add Beans: Add beans to the cooked veggies, mix together until beans are warm.

Spoon bean and veggie mixture into tortillas. Enjoy!

TIP:

Top with **Cashew Sour Cream**. Combine 1 cup of soaked cashews with 1/2 cup water, 1 tablespoon lemon juice, 1 teaspoon apple cider vinegar, and 1/2 teaspoon salt in a high speed blender. Blend until smooth.

9
THINK EXERCISE

Brain Health

"Your shirt has more wrinkles than I do," Maxine says to her teenage grandson as he sits down at the table for breakfast.

"Yeah, no one cares, Grams." Despite his aloof demeanor, Malik secretly enjoys her witty humor.

"Well, change my name to No One." She chuckles. "If I showed up at the museum like that, they'd send me home. Or to a home."

Malik is staying with his grandparents for two weeks while he participates in an internship program at the local hospital where students are researching dementia.

Maxine drops Malik off at the hospital on her way to work, where she arranges flowers at a historic home. She recently announced her retirement because she felt slow compared to the other employees, but her boss refused to accept it, citing the value of her accumulated wisdom.

After years of visiting her mother in a memory care unit, Maxine explains her fear of lying in a bed while her family visits with photo albums. "Do you ever worry about that?" she asks her coworker, Jane, who is the second oldest in the group.

"Sometimes, but it's out of my control, and I try not to waste time on it." Jane selects a large vase for the front table where guests enter.

"Malik says we're not powerless." Maxine chooses some large blooms for the focal point and places them in the vase.

"You mean we can prevent memory loss?" Jane adds some smaller flowers to fill the vase.

"To some degree, with nutrition and exercise," Maxine says.

Jane interrupts, "That's the answer to everything. I eat a lot of fruits and vegetables, I try to avoid fatty foods, and I rarely eat processed foods. But at my age, isn't it too late to start exercising?"

"The main thing is to keep your body moving. My daughter-in-law, Marta, says all my years of digging and planting shrubs should help. Gardening is a Blue Zone behavior," Maxine beams.

"What's a Blue Zone?"

"They're places in the world where people live longer without all the pills and procedures of modern medicine. People in the Blue Zones are more active and maintain strength and balance into their eighties and nineties.

"Marta explained gardening uses my whole body. Shoveling and squatting are complex movements meaning they use a lot of muscles at the same time. This creates more pathways from the brain to the muscles. Those are the types of movements that benefit us the most." Maxine adds some greenery to support the stems.

Jane pulls one of the taller flowers out and trims the stem. "My daughter, Julia, joined Fabulous Fitness and tried to get me to go with her. She said I should do high-intensity exercise; she called it 'hit.' Do you know anything about that?"

"No, but I'll ask Malik." They finish their work for the day, and Maxine drives back to the hospital.

"How was your day?" Maxine asks Malik as he gets into the car.

"Fine."

"Jane asked me about the 'hit' exercise. Do you know what that is?" She turns her blinker on as she approaches the smoothie shop.

"Yeah, it's pretty cool for brain health. It's an acronym—H-I-I-T—and it stands for High-Intensity Interval Training. It involves exercising at a high intensity for short periods, and there's a lot of science behind it. High intensity causes some brain cells—called glial cells—to convert glucose into lactate. Lactate is used by other brain cells for energy. The process is called the lactate shuttle, and it's believed to be a critical part of learning and memory." Maxine and Malik are waiting to place their order, and Malik raises his voice above the blender noise.

"Lactate also protects the brain because it's anti-inflammatory. The research team is looking at ways to take advantage of this lactate to treat disease."

"So, does high-intensity exercise lower the chance of developing dementia?" Maxine puts a straw in her cup and takes a sip.

"Early research supports that hypothesis, but we need to do more work to determine the perfect balance of intensity and time. There's usually a sweet spot for this type of thing. Not too much, not too little, but just right, like Goldilocks.

"Let's hope the answer is high effort for short periods like when you push a wheelbarrow full of mulch up a hill." Malik hunches his back and grabs the imaginary handles as he lets out a theatrical grunt.

Maxine shakes her head and smiles, "You'd be a lot more convincing if you wiped that smirk off your face."

The next day in the lab, Malik talks to his mentor, Dr. Graymatter. "I was telling my grandmother about the lactate shuttle last night, and she thought lactate was a waste product."

"That was the thinking until we figured out it has a beneficial role in metabolism. Did you also tell her about BDNF—brain-derived neurotrophic factor? It was part of last week's lecture." Dr. Graymatter hopes her students absorb all the details from her presentations.

"I remember we pump out more BDNF at high intensities. The study you mentioned used short bursts of exercise on a stationary bike to show improvements in learning and memory," Malik recalls.

"Those cognitive benefits can happen by increasing BDNF through other activities in addition to exercise. Engaging in new and challenging tasks can boost BDNF." Malik's mentor pulls the tea bag out of her mug and places it in the trash bin.

Dr. Graymatter continues, "And then, of course, don't forget nutrition. Foods like blueberries and green tea that are rich in polyphenols support BDNF production." She takes a sip.

Think Exercise

Jane arrives at the pumpkin patch at the same time as her daughter, Julia. Julia's kids, Jesse and Janine, jump out of their mom's car, run to hug Jane, and then sprint away to explore the corn maze.

"Have you seen the new information about estrogen supplementation? Should I be taking it to prevent dementia?" Jane asks.

Julia has discussed this topic with her colleagues at the Women's Health Center, but the information is inconclusive. "Some studies show if you start it early enough, estrogen may be protective for the brain. But there might be an increased risk of dementia if it's started too late.

"And there are other factors to consider," she continues, "like cardiovascular health and cancer history. I can imagine every doctor needs to make those recommendations on a case-by-case basis."

Julia links arms with her mom as they enter the maze. "Focus on the strategies we know are helpful. What are you having for dinner tonight?"

"Whatever you're cooking," her mom jokes.

Julia smiles. "I put lentil chili in the slow cooker this morning."

SLOW COOKER LENTIL CHILI

PREP TIME: 15 MINUTES   SERVES: 8

INGREDIENTS:

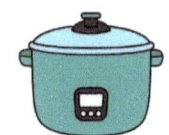

1 medium onion diced

4 cloves garlic minced

2 red peppers chopped

1 green pepper chopped (optional)

3 large carrots diced

3 cups vegetable broth

1 can tomato sauce (15 ounces)

2 cans diced tomatoes (or one 28 ounce can)

1 pound brown lentils rinsed (16 ounces)

2 cans small red beans rinsed and drained (or 3.5 cups)

3 Tablespoon chili powder

1 Tablespoon cumin

Salt and black pepper to taste

DIRECTIONS:

Place all ingredients in a slow cooker (6 quart).

Stir well to combine.

Cover and cook on High for 4-6 hours or low for 8-10 hours.

Serve warm.

NOTES:

The small red beans are a good size to pair with the lentils. You can swap for another bean, but keep in mind that the size of some beans (ex., kidney) will overwhelm the lentils.

Also, this chili freezes well, so it's a great way to make dinner for the future!

10
HOT FLASHES AND HEART DISEASE

Cardiovascular Health

Charlene is on her way to school for parent-teacher conferences before meeting with new clients this afternoon. She feels unstoppable in her favorite skirt with matching tights and a turtleneck sweater. Her winter coat is draped over the passenger seat.

Singing along to the radio, Charlene starts to feel warm. She turns off the heat, then puts on the air conditioning, and finally opens the window.

At 46, Charlene knows hot flashes are a symptom of menopause, but today's flash is intense. "Ugh!" she groans. Her legs are on fire. She approaches a traffic light and prays it stays red. She quickly pulls up the emergency brake and rips the tights off her legs.

Charlene arrives at the school and goes to the bathroom to splash cold water on her face and neck and remove the shredded tights. After the conferences, she leaves school and meets with the new clients, her confidence diminished by the ramifications of the hot flash.

She goes home to change her clothes and heads to the park to meet Gina. "I was at the stoplight near the coffee shop, just a few blocks from school." Charlene relays all the details as she and Gina walk along a path.

"Oh, that's terrible," Gina replies sympathetically.

"Have you ever had a hot flash?" Charlene asks.

"I get small waves of heat, but nothing like that. Remember when we made those plant-based meals a few years ago to help with Carl's diabetes?"

"Yeah," she mumbles as she gives Gina that *here she goes again* look.

"I know. I always talk about food. But hear me out. There was a study with women who had two or more moderate to severe hot flashes every day. The women were divided into two groups, and one group ate low-fat plant-based foods for twelve weeks, including a half-cup of soybeans daily. The other group just continued with their normal diet."

"I bet I can guess the results," Charlene says.

"An eighty-four percent decrease in hot flashes for the women who ate plant-based foods! Isn't that amazing?" Gina exclaims as she watches her friend process the information.

"Wow—that's probably as good as taking hormones. How does food help with hot flashes?"

"Isoflavones in soy can mimic estrogen by interacting with estrogen receptors, which is especially helpful when estrogen levels decline during menopause. Plus, the fiber in plant-based foods supports a healthier gut microbiome, and certain gut bacteria can convert these compounds into forms that help reduce menopausal symptoms. This may be why women in cultures that consume more soy products often report fewer hot flashes than women in the U.S."

Gina continues, "The research also showed the women eating plant-based foods lost almost eight pounds during the twelve weeks, and they had significant changes in their microbiome—the bacteria living in the intestines. Some of the bacteria associated with heart disease, type 2 diabetes, and rheumatoid arthritis died off."

A few days later, Gina joins her father and Aunt Ginger at their retirement community for lunch. In the freshly decorated dining room, dozens of residents sit at tables eating the featured dish of the day.

"They serve fried chicken every Tuesday," Ginger says. "It's one of the best meals they make. You should try it!"

Gina politely declines and orders a side salad with a baked potato and broccoli. Toward the end of the meal, Ginger rubs her left shoulder and complains of indigestion. "I'll get an antacid when I get back to my apartment," she says.

That night, Ginger vomits and has episodes of diarrhea. She assumes it was something she ate, which it was, just not in the way she imagines. Instead of acute food poisoning, Ginger's symptoms are the result of *chronic* food poisoning.

In the morning, Ginger asks one of the nurses for something she can take to feel better. As she describes her symptoms, the nurse alerts the staff doctor. Ginger is taken to the emergency room to rule out a heart attack. Several hours later, she is admitted to the hospital, and two stents are placed in the arteries around her heart to restore blood flow.

"No one thought she was having a heart attack because she didn't have chest pain," Gina tells Charlene on the phone later that day. "She said it was heartburn."

"What made the nurse think it might be a heart attack?" Charlene wonders aloud.

"Nurses are trained to recognize the uncommon symptoms of heart disease like pain in the neck or shoulder, and sometimes the jaw. Vomiting is another clue so they knew it was worth evaluating.

"Did you know heart disease is the leading cause of death for men *and* women?" Gina asks. "For women, the risk increases as estrogen declines. As much as we worry about breast cancer, heart disease is a bigger risk. Twice as many women die from heart disease than all forms of cancer combined."

"How does estrogen protect against heart disease?"

"Estrogen is an antioxidant, and it fights inflammation, so it has a protective effect on blood vessels. Without it, we need to focus on other ways to take care of our cardiovascular system."

"Like what?" Charlene asks.

"Eating foods high in antioxidants is one way. Vitamin C, Vitamin E, and beta-carotene are antioxidants, and good sources are broccoli, sweet potatoes, leafy greens, avocados, lemons and oranges, and bell peppers. Most fruits and vegetables contain antioxidants."

Here are some good sources of antioxidants!

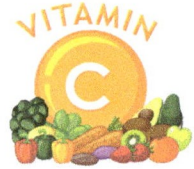

Pineapple – 79 mg/cup (100% DRI)
Mango – 60 mg/cup (80% DRI)
Red Bell Peppers – 190 mg/cup chopped (over 250% DRI)
Strawberries – 98 mg/cup (over 100% DRI)
Oranges – 70 mg per medium orange (almost 100% DRI)

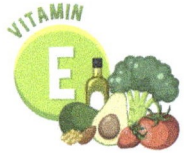

Sunflower Seeds – 7.4 mg per 1 ounce (49% DRI)
Almonds – 7.3 mg per 1 ounce (48% DRI)
Spinach – 3.7 mg per 1 cup cooked (25% DRI)
Avocado – 2.7 mg per 1 avocado (18% DRI)
Hazelnuts – 4.3 mg per 1 ounce (29% DRI)

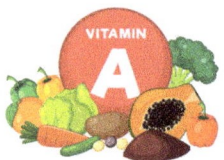

Sweet Potatoes – 11,000 mcg/cup cooked (over 100% DRI)
Carrots – 9,000 mcg/cup raw (about 100% DRI)
Butternut Squash – 9,500 mcg/cup cooked (over 100% DRI)
Kale – 6,000 mcg/cup cooked (about 70% DRI)
Cantaloupe – 3,000 mcg/cup (about 35% DRI)

mg = milligrams, mcg = micrograms, DRI = daily recommended intake

"Can't I just take a multivitamin?"

"Vitamins and minerals work better when we eat them in combination with the other nutrients in the plants. Supplements don't provide the same benefits."

Ginger is released from the hospital and returns to the retirement community. She makes time to talk to the nurses about how to reduce her risk of another heart attack.

Ginger touches the wrinkles over her top lip. "I stopped smoking a few years ago. But I probably smoked a pack a day for over thirty years. What else can I do?"

"Not smoking is a great start. But I can't stress enough how important food and exercise are for a healthy heart. Focus on foods low in saturated fat and high in fiber to improve cholesterol and triglycerides. And keep your body moving," Nurse Nancy advises as she untangles the cords on the portable blood pressure monitor.

"I eat here, so I assume my diet is good. But I'll cut back on the fried chicken I was eating when this all started. Usually, I eat yogurt for breakfast, tuna and cottage cheese for lunch, and maybe a piece of chicken or fish for dinner," Ginger says.

"What about foods with fiber?" Nancy points to the chart at the nurses' station that encourages twenty-five to thirty grams of fiber per day.

Ginger looks puzzled, and the nurse continues.

"Fiber is important to get rid of excess cholesterol in the body. Plants are the only natural source of fiber, so we need to eat plant foods at each meal. The only research studies that have shown reversal of heart disease, where the plaque in the arteries actually gets smaller, used plant-based foods."

Ginger responds with a scrunched face, "I don't care for vegetables."

"You can't hate all vegetables. Try adding a fruit or vegetable, or some beans or whole grains, to one meal a day," Nancy suggests. "Not only will you reduce your risk of another heart attack, but you'll also reduce your risk of breast cancer, dementia, and plenty of other conditions."

"It's certainly a good incentive." Ginger turns and walks toward the lounge to get an apple.

ANTIOXIDANT SOUP

SERVES: 4-6   PREP TIME: 30 MINUTES

INGREDIENTS:

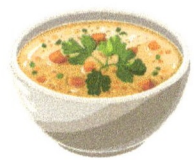

1 onion, diced
3 tablespoons garlic, minced
2 tablespoons ginger, minced
3 carrots, chopped
1-2 sweet potatoes, chopped (about 2 cups)
1 teaspoon dried turmeric
3/4 cup dried red lentils
1/2 teaspoon salt
4 cups vegetable broth
2 cups kale or spinach, chopped
1 lemon, juiced

DIRECTIONS:

Saute: In a large pot over medium heat, saute onion and garlic in water for 3-5 minutes. Add carrots and sweet potatoes, saute for 5 more minutes. Add turmeric and ginger, saute for another minute.

Cook Lentils: Add broth, lentils, and salt. Stir and bring to a boil. Reduce heat and simmer for 10-15 minutes.

Remove from heat and stir in greens and lemon juice. After a few minutes, greens will wilt. Serve and Enjoy!

TIP:

Sourdough bread would pair nicely with this soup.

11
PINK FOR PREVENTION

Breast Health

"Are you coming Saturday?" Beth unloads the water bottle and sunscreen from the heap in her friend's arms.

"To what?" Tasha sets up her stadium seat on the bleachers.

"The breast cancer walk. It's a 5K, and most of us will be there." Beth looks around at the women watching the baseball game.

"Yeah, I'll walk, but with all the money being used to find a cure, wouldn't it be nice if more of the research could focus on prevention? Seems like we should try to keep cancer from developing in the first place."

Tasha continues, "Just last week, drum lines from local schools played at a rally to raise awareness about breast cancer prevention. It was pretty cool." The crowd stands and cheers when the center fielder catches a fly ball at the wall.

"Are there ways to prevent breast cancer?" Beth considers this idea.

"Organizers at the rally handed out fliers about using a four-pronged approach for prevention: eat plant-based foods, exercise, maintain a healthy weight, and limit alcohol." Tasha counts each one on her hand as she lists them.

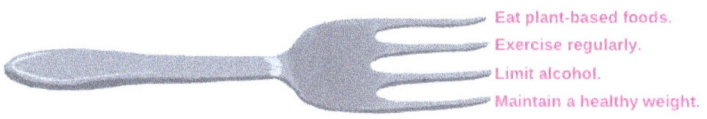

"What even is a healthy weight?" Beth asks, knowing there is so much controversy over this topic.

"For the research data, they used BMI—body mass index—which you can calculate from your height and weight. It's a decent measurement to use as a reference point."

The crowd jumps up as Beth's son hits a double into left field. "Keep those bats going!" Tasha hollers as she sits back down.

Tasha continues, "Too much body fat increases the chances of developing breast cancer, especially after menopause. And extra fat makes cancer more likely to spread. Fat cells produce a form of estrogen that binds to the receptors on cancer cells and helps them grow."

Beth takes a sip of water as she thinks about the bottle of wine she splits with her husband every night. "And what about alcohol?"

"Unfortunately, even one drink a day increases the risk of breast cancer regardless of whether it's beer or wine or liquor. Alcohol causes DNA damage, which is the first step in the development of cancer cells."

Tasha scrolls through her photos and shows Beth a picture of a mango-colored beverage in a martini glass. "I was at a happy hour with my mother-in-law recently, and the bar served mocktails. I got a Seaside Sipper, and it was excellent!"

Beth rolls her eyes at the suggestion but takes it into consideration. "And how do plant-based foods help reduce the risk of breast cancer?"

"A couple of ways. One, plants are high in fiber and other nutrients, which help the body get rid of cancer-causing chemicals. Adding soy-based foods can also lower your risk. And you can also decrease your risk by avoiding processed meats like bacon and sausage."

The crowd roars. Tasha and Beth jump to their feet as the umpire shouts and pumps his fist across his body, "Strike Three! You're out."

A few months later, Tasha sees her gynecologist for her annual appointment. While the doctor reviews her mammogram results, Tasha describes a recent change. "My breasts are more tender. Is that anything to worry about?"

Dr. Bloom explains, "Your mammogram looks good, but you're in perimenopause, and the fluctuating estrogen level can cause tenderness. Just keep up with your annual breast cancer screening.

"The risk of breast cancer increases with age, especially after menopause. Eight out of ten cases of breast cancer are women over fifty."

"I can reduce my risk with lifestyle changes, right?" Tasha is looking for confirmation of the four-pronged approach.

"Absolutely!" Dr. Bloom is excited when patients want to participate in keeping themselves healthy. She hands Tasha a patient brochure that includes beautiful plant-based recipes.

"Anything I can do about this?" Tasha cups her hands under her breasts.

"If your weight increases, fat stores in the breast tissue grow, putting strain on the ligaments, which contributes to saggy breasts. But more importantly, it's harder to diagnose breast cancer because it's more difficult to find lumps."

"Even more reason to keep my weight in a reasonable range," Tasha mutters.

DANDY COCOA LATTE

SERVES: 1   PREP TIME: 5 MINUTES

Without the caffeine from coffee, this is a great alternative for a latte anytime of day.

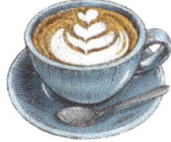

INGREDIENTS:

1 cup unsweetened vanilla soy milk (or oat milk)
1 tablespoon cocoa powder
1 tablespoon Dandy Blend
1 tablespoon maple syrup

DIRECTIONS:

Combine ingredients in a glass measuring cup that holds 2 cups or more of liquid. Using an immersion blender (or a whisk), mix together. (I prefer the immersion blender to create froth.)

Pour into a mug or insulated cup and enjoy!

TIP:

Add 1/2 teaspoon of cinnamon for additional flavor and the health benefits. Cinnamon is an antioxidant and anti-inflammatory, it improves insulin sensitivity, and promotes gut health.

12
ESTROGEN AFFECTS EVERYTHING

Not So Obvious

The women arrive at one o'clock on Sunday for their monthly book club meeting. Anya greets them at the door and leads them to the family room, where the fire is crackling.

Susan sits in a chair near the hearth and Lisa curls up in the corner of the sofa. Debra sits on the other end and notices Susan covering her ear with her hand. "Shoot, my ear is ringing."

"From what?" Debra asks.

"I had coffee at brunch and probably forgot to order decaf. It makes my tinnitus worse." Susan has complained about her condition for the past few years.

Lisa sits up straighter. "My friend had tinnitus during perimenopause, and her doctor gave her estrogen therapy. I think the ringing stopped."

"How did estrogen help?" Susan asks.

"She said it regulates the fluid balance in the inner ear. During menopause, the lack of estrogen can disrupt that balance and cause ringing or humming in the ear. There are other causes of tinnitus, but it's worth looking into."

"Huh, I'll ask my doctor. Thanks." Susan sets a reminder on her phone to message her doctor.

Later, the women drift from the book discussion back to health issues.

Debra, who has been complaining of fatigue for months, updates the group. "I had blood work done and started on thyroid medicine a few weeks ago. I feel a little better. My doctor said an underactive thyroid is common in women during menopause."

"My thyroid levels were low too. My doctor told me not to skip breakfast, especially when I go to the gym. He's going to recheck in a few weeks." Anya shrugs her shoulders, expressing her skepticism of this approach. "I do have more energy, for what it's worth."

"How can eating breakfast help your thyroid?" Debra hates taking medicine and would love to try anything else.

"Evidently, when the body senses less energy is available, the brain sends a signal to the thyroid gland to slow things down. The thyroid makes less of its hormones, T3 and T4."

"Interesting," Debra says. "I've always thought of low thyroid as the problem, not the response to another issue."

Anya replies, "It kind of makes sense that the body can regulate thyroid hormone levels based on the availability of food. It's like your body is switching into power-saving mode, the way your phone dims its screen and slows performance when the battery is low. It's just trying to stretch the energy it has."

Finding a Balance

Healthy eating and exercise can pose a challenge for many women, especially as they enter perimenopause and experience changes in their body composition. If the body senses a relative energy deficiency, it finds ways to conserve energy, like dialing down thyroid hormone.

Energy deficiency manifests as fatigue, hunger, trouble sleeping, and waking up hungry in the middle of the night. It can also show up as delayed healing, increased susceptibility to infections, and mental health issues like irritability, anxiety, and depression.

To lose fat and gain strength, eat most of your calories at breakfast, lunch, and mid-afternoon, and minimize calories in the evening by eating a small dinner with lower caloric density foods. Eat when your body needs fuel during the active times of the day, and let the body recover and repair during sleep without needing to digest food.

"My doctor thinks my fatigue is from insulin resistance," Lisa offers.

Susan is sympathetic. "As in diabetes?"

"Not quite, but I'm pre-diabetic. She told me we're more insulin-resistant as we go through menopause."

"What did she recommend?" Susan thinks of her sister, who struggles to keep her blood sugar under control.

Lisa sighs. "Exercise. She says walking after meals will be helpful. I need to figure out a way to make this a priority."

> ### Trouble opening a jar?
>
> A study of more than 4,000 postmenopausal women aged 45 to 65 found that weaker grip strength is associated with a greater likelihood of having diabetes. Grip strength is a proxy for muscle, and less muscle mass is linked to higher odds of diabetes. Strength training the whole body will build and preserve lean muscle tissue.

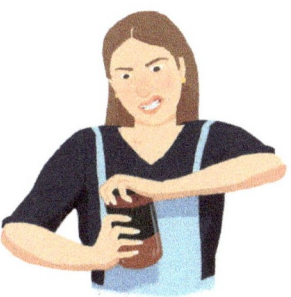

"Maybe we can work on this stuff together. We're all in some stage of menopause. We can help each other with accountability. When we get together each month, we can dedicate some of the time to talk about anything new we learn." Anya pauses to assess their reaction.

With no objections, Anya adds, "Okay, then. Next month we'll talk about our book and check in on what exercise routines everyone is doing. We may be at different stages, but we can all provide support."

"I wonder how other mammals deal with menopause," Lisa asks.

"Actually, only humans, orcas, and a few other mammals live past reproductive age. And remember the life expectancy of a woman in developed countries in 1900 was only forty-eight. It's relatively new territory."

Bottom Line

Although menopause is technically a specific day in time, it's also an ongoing journey. By incorporating lifestyle changes—through nutrition, exercise, sleep, and stress management—women can be proactive about the future.

Small, consistent efforts in the following areas can help you maintain a vibrant, fulfilling lifestyle for years to come.

Exercise

- Stay active.
- Strength train to reclaim muscle and bone loss.
- Work near maximal effort during short bursts of cardiovascular training.
- Perform balance exercises to prevent falls and jumping exercises to strengthen bones.

Nutrition

- Eat whole plant foods to maximize the anti-inflammatory effects, feed the gut microbiome, and stimulate the production of mood-boosting compounds.

Sleep

- Develop a routine with a consistent bedtime.
- Practice sleep hygiene (limit screens, alcohol, and food before bed).

Stress Management

- Reduce stress by talking to friends, volunteering, journaling, or enjoying other activities that bring you joy.
- Make time to recover and relax.

If you want additional support, don't delay in seeking help from your doctor, a menopause specialist, or another trusted healthcare provider. Combinations of therapies are warranted when trying to achieve optimal outcomes.

Here's to outsmarting menopause!

Brooke

Frequently Asked Questions about Estrogen Supplementation

Q: Should I take hormone replacement therapy (HRT)?
A: Talk to your healthcare provider to determine the risks and benefits for you. There are many factors to consider, and a conversation with your healthcare provider is imperative.

Q: Why don't all women take hormones after menopause?
A: Some women experience side effects. They may be mild, like vaginal bleeding, but they could be more serious such as blood clots and cancer.

Q: Is MHT the same as HRT?
A: MHT, Menopause Hormone Therapy, has a narrower focus for treating the symptoms of menopause with estrogen and progesterone. Even though the terms are used interchangeably, HRT, Hormone Replacement Therapy, is used more broadly to replace estrogen in a variety of estrogen-deficient conditions.

Q: How are oral contraceptives different from HRT or MHT?
A: The hormones in oral contraceptive pills are present in much higher doses than HRT or MHT. The purpose of oral contraceptives is to shut down ovulation to prevent pregnancy. This type of birth control is prescribed for younger women, but after the age of 35, the risk of blood clots, heart attacks, strokes, and breast cancer increases with these higher doses of hormones.

ANTI-INFLAMMATORY CHICKPEAS AND GREENS

SERVES: 2   PREP TIME: 10 MINUTES

INGREDIENTS:

1 can (15.5 ounces) chickpeas, drained and rinsed
1 can (14.5 ounces) diced tomatoes, not drained
1 teaspoon cumin
1 teaspoon chili powder
1/2 teaspoon salt
1/4 teaspoon black pepper
1/4 teaspoon garlic powder
1-2 handfuls of spinach or kale, finely chopped

DIRECTIONS:

Combine Ingredients: Add all ingredients to a bowl (for the no-cook version), a pot (for stovetop cooking), or a microwave-safe dish (for microwave preparation) and stir well.

For the no-cook version, serve and enjoy.

For the stovetop version, cook mixture until greens wilt and contents reach desired temperature, about 5 minutes.

For the microwave version, cook mixture until greens wilt and contents reach desired temperature, about 3 minutes.

TIP:

This recipe is on the Quick Cooks App!

Author's Note

Dear Reader,

I hope you gained new insights about menopause and feel empowered by the knowledge. I'd be grateful if you would take the time to leave a review on Amazon. Your feedback not only helps me as an author but also guides others to find a helpful resource. Together, we can navigate menopause with strength and confidence!

Stay strong, and be well!

Brooke

BRAIN-BOOSTING BLONDIES

SERVES: 2   PREP TIME: 10 MINUTES

INGREDIENTS:

1 can (15.5 ounces) chickpeas, drained and rinsed
1/2 cup peanut butter
1/3 cup maple syrup
2 teaspoons vanilla
1/2 teaspoon salt
1/4 teaspoon baking powder
1/4 teaspoon baking soda
1/4 cup chopped walnuts
1/4 cup dairy-free chocolate chips

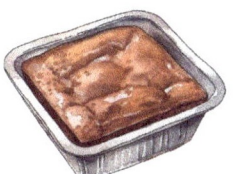

DIRECTIONS:

Prepare Oven and Pan: Preheat oven to 350 degrees F and line an 8x8 pan with parchment paper.

Combine Ingredients: In a food processor, add all ingredients except walnuts and chocolate chips. Process until batter is smooth. Fold in walnuts and chocolate chips.

Spread batter into pan and bake for 20-25 minutes. Use a toothpick to check the blondies; it should come out clean. Be careful not to overcook or they will be too dry. (If that happens, use as a topping on a smoothie bowl.)

TIP:

This batter can be eaten without cooking.

About the Author

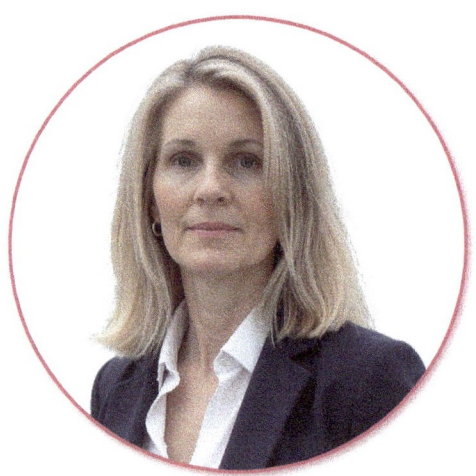

Swapping her white coat for an apron and her stethoscope for a dumbbell, Dr. Brooke Bussard believes in the power of nutrition and lifestyle for optimal health.

With the goal of preventing and reversing the chronic conditions associated with aging, Brooke enjoys watching people improve their health by implementing behaviors that fit into their daily lives.

When she is not gardening with her husband, spending time with their sons, or hiking with friends, Brooke enjoys speaking to all age groups about the powerful link between food, fitness, and good health.

A graduate of the University of Virginia's School of Medicine and College of Arts & Sciences, Brooke blends her medical knowledge with her expertise in fitness and nutrition.

CARROT CAKE SMOOTHIE

SERVES: 1   PREP TIME: 5 MINUTES

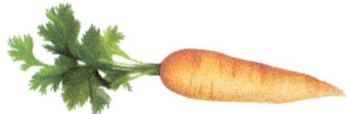

INGREDIENTS:

1 frozen banana
½ cup carrots (about 1 medium carrot)
1 cup oat or soy milk (unsweetened or vanilla)
1 tablespoon peanut butter (smooth or crunchy)
½ teaspoon ground cinnamon
¼ teaspoon ground nutmeg
    (optional, for extra carrot cake flavor)
1 teaspoon maple syrup (optional, for sweetness)
1 tablespoon rolled oats (optional, for a thicker smoothie)
Handful of ice cubes (optional, for a colder smoothie)

DIRECTIONS:

Combine: In a blender, combine the banana, grated carrots, oat milk, peanut butter, cinnamon, nutmeg (if using), and maple syrup (if desired). Add rolled oats for extra thickness and ice cubes for a colder smoothie, if you prefer.

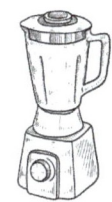

Blend Until Smooth: Blend on high speed until smooth and creamy.

Serve: Pour into a glass, sprinkle with a pinch of cinnamon on top, and enjoy immediately!

Contributors

This book is the result of not just my own efforts but also the invaluable insights, feedback, and encouragement from a wonderful group of individuals who generously shared their time and perspectives. As beta readers, these contributors played a crucial role in shaping the final version of this book, helping to refine its ideas, clarify its messages, and ensure its relevance and impact. Their honesty, thoughtful critiques, and encouragement are true gifts, and I am deeply grateful for their contributions. Listed here are the names of those who were part of this collaborative journey—thank you for helping make this book the best it can be!

Tracy Immerman Cioni
Monica Goldstone
Naomi Shapiro
Kathy Eades
Patsy Bussard
Betty H. Kansler
Kim Seaney
Melissa Schechter
Melissa Kaplan
Debra Shapiro, M.D., FACOG

www.ingramcontent.com/pod-product-compliance
Lightning Source LLC
Chambersburg PA
CBHW052033030426
42337CB00027B/4980